T0275638

CAMBRIDGE LIBRARY COLLECTION

Books of enduring scholarly value

History of Medicine

It is sobering to realise that as recently as the year in which On the Origin of Species was published, learned opinion was that diseases such as typhus and cholera were spread by a 'miasma', and suggestions that doctors should wash their hands before examining patients were greeted with mockery by the profession. The Cambridge Library Collection reissues milestone publications in the history of Western medicine as well as studies of other medical traditions. Its coverage ranges from Galen on anatomical procedures to Florence Nightingale's common-sense advice to nurses, and includes early research into genetics and mental health, colonial reports on tropical diseases, documents on public health and military medicine, and publications on spa culture and medicinal plants.

The Soldier's Manual of Sanitation

This joint reissue comprises two works on military medicine, providing instruction on the treatment of ailments common to soldiers, and methods for preventing their occurrence. The title work, written by Charles Alexander Gordon (1821–99) and published in 1873, is followed by *A Guide to Health for the Use of Soldiers* by fellow surgeon R.C. Eaton (1842–1902), which first appeared in 1890. Intended to be read by infantrymen and officers, both works offer succinct and practical advice on topics ranging from malaria to drunkenness. The texts take slightly different approaches in their presentation of advice: Gordon adopts a crisp and formal style, while Eaton incorporates instructive medical facts in his brief yet fluent explanations. Together, the works provide an effective exposition of problems and practicalities that would assume tremendous significance decades later in the trenches of the First World War.

Cambridge University Press has long been a pioneer in the reissuing of out-of-print titles from its own backlist, producing digital reprints of books that are still sought after by scholars and students but could not be reprinted economically using traditional technology. The Cambridge Library Collection extends this activity to a wider range of books which are still of importance to researchers and professionals, either for the source material they contain, or as landmarks in the history of their academic discipline.

Drawing from the world-renowned collections in the Cambridge University Library and other partner libraries, and guided by the advice of experts in each subject area, Cambridge University Press is using state-of-the-art scanning machines in its own Printing House to capture the content of each book selected for inclusion. The files are processed to give a consistently clear, crisp image, and the books finished to the high quality standard for which the Press is recognised around the world. The latest print-on-demand technology ensures that the books will remain available indefinitely, and that orders for single or multiple copies can quickly be supplied.

The Cambridge Library Collection brings back to life books of enduring scholarly value (including out-of-copyright works originally issued by other publishers) across a wide range of disciplines in the humanities and social sciences and in science and technology.

The Soldier's Manual of Sanitation

And of First Help in Sickness and when Wounded

C͏HARLES A͏LEXANDER G͏ORDON

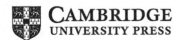

CAMBRIDGE
UNIVERSITY PRESS

University Printing House, Cambridge, CB2 8BS, United Kingdom

Published in the United States of America by Cambridge University Press, New York

Cambridge University Press is part of the University of Cambridge.
It furthers the University's mission by disseminating knowledge in the pursuit of
education, learning and research at the highest international levels of excellence.

www.cambridge.org
Information on this title: www.cambridge.org/9781108069885

© in this compilation Cambridge University Press 2014

This edition first published 1873
This digitally printed version 2014

ISBN 978-1-108-06988-5 Paperback

THE SOLDIER'S
MANUAL OF SANITATION

AND OF

First Help in Sickness and when Wounded.

ADAPTED FOR

OFFICERS, NON-COMMISSIONED OFFICERS, AND PRIVATES
OF THE ACTIVE FORCES,
MILITIA, YEOMANRY, AND VOLUNTEERS, FOR HOME
AND FOREIGN SERVICE,

FOR PEACE AND FOR WAR.

By DEPUTY SURGEON-GENERAL
CHARLES ALEXANDER GORDON, M.D., C.B.

———

" Mon bien le plus précieux, c'est la santé du soldat.'
TURENNE.

———

LONDON:
BAILLIERE, TINDALL, & COX,
KING WILLIAM STREET, STRAND.
———
1873.

LONDON:

PRINTED BY BAILLIERE, TINDALL, AND COX.

KING WILLIAM STREET, STRAND.

INTRODUCTORY.

MANUALS of various kinds, specially intended for use by the soldier, are published in the several countries of Europe, and among them instructions given, more or less detailed, in regard to the best means of preserving health, decreasing the risks of sickness, and of affording some measure of aid to their comrades when attacked by illness or wounded in battle. I have accordingly been induced to frame the following brief directions, in the hope that they may reach the hands of non-commissioned officers and private soldiers in our own army, whether of the active or auxiliary services. I have endeavoured to adapt them to the varying conditions of our army, and it only remains to be seen how far they may be considered useful to those for whom they are particularly intended.

C. A. GORDON.

April, 1873.

THE SOLDIER'S

MANUAL OF SANITATION

ACCIDENT.—A soldier has fallen, say from a height or down a stair. He is found at the foot, severely injured and insensible. At first it is impossible to say what is the nature or extent of his injuries, but his limbs are doubled up underneath him, and he is bleeding from the head or other part. In such a case, the first care of the man who first finds him should be to deal gently with him, for the chances are that a limb, or a rib, or perhaps more than one, are broken. He should therefore be carefully and, without roughness, turned over and placed in a natural position, his limbs stretched out, his collar and tunic undone. He is better placed upon his back than in any other position, as on it he can breathe most easily, and water can best be thrown upon his face. If his limbs are bent in other parts than at the joints they are *broken;* and in that case require the greatest care in being brought back into position. If they cannot be naturally moved at the joints, they are *dislocated.* If a second man be present, he should be sent for a stretcher, and the injured one conveyed to hospital.—*See* STRETCHERS.

ACCOMMODATION.—The nature of the accommodation afforded to troops exercises an important influence upon their health. Under ordinary circumstances soldiers occupy only such buildings and places as have been selected with great care for them ; on active service, however, and occasionally also under other conditions, neither the soldiers nor their officers are in a position to select their accommodation, it may therefore be of some importance to them to have a few general instructions on this point. It is a principle of army hygiene that the *accommodation* of the soldier has an importance equal to that possessed by his clothing and food, and it is known that certain diseases, more especially those of the chest, as well as some kinds of fever, are produced or averted according to the way in which men are housed. Whatever be the kind of accommodation, there are three requirements that must be considered, namely—space, ventilation, and cleanliness. These are necessary to health, and it were better that men should sleep in the open air, with no other covering than their great coats and blankets, than be *accommodated* in buildings where these requirements are non-attainable. On active service, the use of buildings usually occupied by crowded assemblies—as churches, theatres, ball-rooms, &c.—should be avoided. When private houses are used temporarily, it is customary to consider that in rooms 15 feet wide, or less, one man for every yard in length may be accommodated ; in those over 15 feet wide, but under 25 feet, two men per yard of length ; for rooms of more than 25 feet broad, three men for every yard in length.—*See* SPACE.

AGUE.—In countries or stations where this affection prevails, *quinine* is now issued to soldiers as a preventive. Experience has quite proved the usefulness of this remedy for the purpose, and therefore soldiers should seek to receive it sufficiently early ; for once that they have actually become attacked with ague, it is, of course, too late for them to take preventive measures—they must then apply to their medical officers. In districts where ague prevails, soldiers should guard themselves as much as possible from exposure at night. When weakened by debauch they are more liable to be attacked by this, and, indeed, all other diseases, than they are while their bodily strength is unimpaired by excesses. Good and plenty of food, sobriety, and suitable clothing are the best means of guarding against ague.—*See* MALARIA.

AIR.—Without pure air around us and to breathe we should speedily become poisoned, as completely so as if we were to imbibe any of the substances known to be destructive of life. Each full-grown healthy man takes into his chest about thirty inches of air at each inspiration, discharging nearly the same quantity, but considerably altered at each expiration. Not only does the air around him become thus *tainted* with the ordinary gaseous products of breathing, but also with the numerous—although invisible—shreds from the lungs, throat, and mouth that are continually being thrown off, and from the perspiration which constantly is going on from the surface of the body, although in too small quantities and too gradually for one to be conscious of it, the total amount being 25 to 40 ounces per day. When men themselves, or their comrades, are not careful of cleanliness, or when they are suffering from disease, the nature of the materials thrown off from them into the air becomes most offensive and injurious to health, and may readily be seen by means of a microscope; thus, then, the necessity of constant change of air in occupied rooms is self-evident. It is calculated that each man in barracks should have a space equal to 600 cubic feet of air in temperate climates, and that of this quantity about 220 should be changed at least every two hours. Men know that in certain states of the air their sensations are different from what they are at others. Damp warm air depresses, while dry air exhilarates. The fear of exposing themselves to the air in barracks is groundless, and it is only those persons who neglect to do so habitually who suffer from "cold," when accidentally exposed to draughts. It is more injurious for men to sleep in foul air than to breathe it during the day or when awake. The risks from foul air increase according with the numbers of men occupying the same place, and the longer time they are continuously together; hence the necessity of leaving occupied rooms absolutely vacant for a certain time daily. Air is also more liable to become foul where vegetation is absent than where it exists in moderate quantity. Dirt, low moral state, ignorance, and prejudice, especially among soldiers' families, result in foulness of air and discomfort in their quarters.

AMUSEMENTS.—Unless the spare time of a soldier can be occupied by amusements in barracks, he will seek for them elsewhere, hence it is that so much has of late years been done to supply him with these. As a rule, however, those most enjoyed are such as are of a muscular nature; rackets, cricket, ball, or quoits, taking the place of the reading-room. This is very natural, and probably it might be well to recognise the fact. Muscular amusements benefit the soldier's health in two important respects: by indulging in them he is kept away from low localities and persons, and his powers are kept in practice for the active duties which form the reasons of his existence as a soldier.

ANATOMY OF A MAN'S BODY.—In general terms a man's body may be described as consisting of a framework formed by bones, covered by flesh or muscles, and enclosed in the skin. The arteries and veins form vessels by which the blood is carried to, and distributed in, the head, trunk, and limbs, and by which after having nourished these various parts it is returned to the heart, whence it again begins its circuit. The *head* comprises the cranium, in which the brains are contained, and the face. The *neck* connects the head with the trunk, and is usually for the sake of convenience considered as belonging more to the former than the latter. The front of the neck is usually spoken of as the throat; the back part, as the nape, forming as it does the upper portion of the back bone, spine or vertebral column. The *trunk* comprises the thorax or chest, abdomen or belly, and the pelvis or lower belly. The chest is formed on either side by the ribs, bent like so many bows. To them the sternum or breast bone is attached in front, and between them behind is the spinal column or back-bone to which they are firmly attached by means of joints admitting of slight motion. At the upper part and in rear of the chest are the shoulder blades, one on either side of the spine, and forming the shoulder. Within the chest are contained the lungs, one on either side by which respiration is performed, and the heart, which beats during life and propels the blood through the various vessels in which it circulates. The precise position of the heart is indicated by the left nipple, and from that point to the pit of the stomach its beat can generally be felt or seen. The abdomen or belly is that part of the trunk situated between the chest and the upper portion of the circle of bone forming the hips and arch of the groin. At the upper and front part is the pit of the stomach or epigastrium, containing the stomach and intestines or bowels; to the right, under the short or false ribs is situated the liver, to the left in the corresponding position, the spleen, behind and on either side of the back bone in the *reins*, are the kidneys, from which the French name of the *region* or division of the body is taken. The *loins* include the space at the back between the short ribs and upper edge of the hip bones, being but another term for the reins. This part is also called the *lumbar* region. The lower belly or pelvis is formed by a solid circle of bone, the sides of which are called the hip bones, the back part the *sacrum* or *sacred* bone, and the front, the pelvis. Within this circle are contained the bladder and part of the great intestine or rectum. This circle gives support at the sides to the thighs by means of the hip joints. In front the *genital* organs are attached; behind and towards the sides are the *buttocks*, and between them, below and in the centre the *anus* or lower opening of the bowels. The limbs comprise the *superior extremities* or arms, and the *inferior* or legs. The superior are united to the chest by the shoulder joint or articulation, the movements of which are the freest of all joints; the limb comprising the arm, fore-arm and hand. The arm consists of only one bone, the fore-arm of two placed side by side; the joint connecting the two parts being the elbow. The hand consists of many bones. It is united to the fore-arm by means of the wrist joint. It comprises the *hand* properly so called, and the fingers, the thumb being anatomically included as a finger. The hand includes the *carpus* and *metacarpus*. The *inferior extremities* or *legs*, are much stronger than the arms. They are all attached to the trunk of the body by means of the hip joints, and include three divisions; namely, the thigh, leg, and foot. The thigh, like the arm, consists of one bone, the leg of two, the joint between those parts being the knee, on the front of which is the knee-cap, or *patella;* behind the *ham*, or *popliteal space.* The front part of the leg is called the *shin;* the part behind, the *calf.* The foot, like the hand, is composed of several bones, these forming the *foot* proper and the *toes.* The foot comprises the *tarsus* and *metatarsus.* It is united to the leg by means of the *ankle*-joint, immediately behind which is the *tendo-Achilles.* The point of support of the foot is at the hinder part, the *heel;* in front, the *ball* of the toes. The part between these points includes the *sole* or *arch* of the foot; the *instep* being the upper or convex part of that arch.

The body is nourished by the *blood.* The blood contains the natural nourishment removed from the food in the process of digestion, the refuse being discharged in the shape of *fœces,* &c. The blood being sent on from the heart, circulates to all parts by means of *arteries,* returning to it by the *veins.* The arteries beat in correspondence with the beat of the heart, and can readily be felt at different points, the wrist being the most usual ; the beat there constituting the pulse. The blood contained in the arteries is of a bright vermillion colour. The *veins* bring back to the heart the blood after it has given its nourishing properties to the different parts of the body, the blood in them being of a dark colour. They are exempt from pulsation; and those upon the surface can be traced as blue lines of greater or smaller size under the skin. It is desirable that soldiers should have at least a general knowledge of the parts which together constitute their own bodies, and accordingly these particulars are given for their guidance.

ANIMALS in, or near barracks, are prohibited by regulations; cows, pigs, goats, poultry, horses and dogs being specially enumerated as those that are not to be kept or permitted to run loose. In some stations, and especially in India, the practice of keeping pets, is to a certain extent, permitted, and is in many instances deserving of encouragement. Not only does it *humanise* a soldier, developing feelings of kindness in him, but experience shows that no actually vicious man is ever fond of *pets*. The very fact, therefore, of such creatures being kept indicates the existence of some of the better feelings of our human nature. The interest taken by a soldier in a pet, and the time occupied in its care, or playing with it fills up a gap that might otherwise be occupied in ways injurious to health and well-being.

APOPLEXY (*see also* HEAT APOPLEXY).—A man complains of severe pain in his head; there is a sense of fullness; he suddenly falls, or becomes insensible; the breathing is slow and *stertorous*, or, in other words, with heavy snoring; the face is flushed, blue, or of otherwise unnatural colour and aspect; the eyes are open and fixed, or staring; the mouth frothy; the limbs paralysed; involuntary passage of the urine and stools; the pulse slow and weak. Often the patient, while suffering from these symptoms, tosses himself from side to side, and every moment manifests the existing danger of death taking place.

In such a case remove at once all encumbrances, undo the clothes, especially at the collar, take off the necktie or stock, undo the braces, open the waistbelt of the trousers, remove the patient to an open place, where the fresh air may freely play upon him, bathe the head and face, sponge the body with cold water, in summer adding to it vinegar or salt to increase its coldness; place a little vinegar, or hartshorn, or smelling salts under the nostrils, rub the legs and soles of the feet, give the patient cold water alone, or with a little spirits, to drink, and take immediate steps to have him carried to hospital.

BAKING.—In India the native bakers have always been adepts at arranging bakeries on the line of march, and preparing bread for the troops. They have iron frame-pieces of ovens provided by the commissariat; these they cover over with wet clay, and soon thus fit up an oven. On home service steam or field ovens are provided, these being drawn by horses. Each such oven is capable of baking 109 loaves of 3 lbs. each in a batch, and admits of four batches being turned out in ten hours. The field ovens, Aldershot pattern, are of sheet iron, and can turn out 150 lbs. of bread at a time. These were used on the Red River Expedition. Arrangements are officially made for supplying troops with baked bread wherever practicable.

BARRACKS.—Whenever troops enter barracks, whether after a severe march or drill, they should partially close the windows, that is, sufficiently to prevent a direct current of cold wind blowing over them. They should dispose of their arms and equipment in a proper manner, and having done so, proceed to undress themselves slowly. If the clothing is wet, it must be changed without delay, dry articles being put on instead. The hands, face, and feet should be bathed in cold or tepid water, or with spirits and water, excoriations being soothed by the use of a little melted suet or lard, for which purpose French soldiers often carry a small supply. The more free ventilation is maintained the more wholesome barrack rooms will be. Fires favour ventilation, but they do harm at night by rendering the places too hot. Generally some windows to leeward may be kept slightly open. Men should themselves be careful that dirt is not allowed to accumulate in presses and on shelves, into or on which it may be the officers are not in the habit of looking. The idea of having their reserve bread or portion of meat put away among dust, or exposed to the emanations of a barrack room is itself very nasty.

The longer each day soldiers are out of the barrack rooms in which they sleep at night the better for their own health. In hot countries arrangements are made so that they may have *day rooms* in which to pass their time while the state of season or weather prevents them from being out of doors.—See *Queen's Regulations.*

BATHING.—The free use of cold or tepid water to the whole surface of the body is not only grateful according to season, but is absolutely necessary for the preservation of health, by removing offensive and impure matters from the pores and surface generally, and preserving the skin in a flaccid state. In the case of men who have not previously been in the habit of bathing some degree of caution is necessary in breaking them in to the custom; but in the case of those habituated, not only is the free use of cold water bearable in cold weather, but it is enjoyable, and, moreover, fortifies the person using it against catching cold and against various diseases. Men reduced in health by dissipated habits or tropical diseases are often injuriously affected by taking a cold bath, whether in the house or outside. The cases of all such should be noted by their sergeants, and the surgeon made acquainted with them. Bathing in rivers is only to be recommended in European or other temperate climates, and in mild weather. In tropical and other hot countries it is objectionable, except, perhaps, during the cold season, but then, what between the risks of quicksands, alligators, &c., the safest way is to warn the men against indulging in it. Under ordinary circumstances, and more especially after the men come off the march or from severe fatigue duties, they should avoid bathing in rivers or lakes. During the prevalence of strong wind, especially if from the north or east, they ought also to refrain from it. A bath in a river or lake should, if possible, not be taken until three hours after breakfast, or when the stomach is empty. When the men are hot they should undress slowly, then go gradually into the water. They ought not to remain longer than a quarter of an hour in the water, and any time beyond twenty minutes is actually injurious to them. On coming out, a man should dry himself as completely as possible, and having done so, should take moderately active exertion. If bathing in the sea, ten minutes is considered sufficiently long to remain in the water.

The Royal Humane Society has issued the following notice:—Avoid bathing within two hours after a meal, or when exhausted by fatigue or from any other cause, or when the body is cooling after perspiration, or altogether in the open air if, after having been a short time in the water, there is a sense of chilliness, with numbness of the hands and feet; but bathe when the body is warm, provided no time is lost in getting into the water. Avoid chilling the body by sitting or standing undressed on the banks or in boats after having been in the water. Avoid remaining too long in the water; leave the water immediately there is the slightest feeling of chilliness. The vigorous and strong may bathe early in the morning on an empty stomach. The young, and those who are weak, had better bathe two or three hours after a meal; the best time for such is from two to three hours after breakfast. Those who are subject to attacks of giddiness or faintness, and those who suffer from palpitation and other sense of discomfort at the heart, should not bathe without first consulting their medical adviser.

BATTLE.—Every soldier (and officer) before going into battle should be provided with a ticket of identification, and with a long strip of bandage, and a piece of linen for use in the event of his being wounded. The continental troops carry the former around the neck, the two latter in the left pocket of their trowsers. As battle is the great object of the existence of a soldier, so it is the gravest duty in which he can be engaged. It is well therefore that men should behave worthily of these two circumstances, with a steady determination to fulfil their duty, whatever the result may be to themselves individually. Great elation of spirits, or great excitement, soon give way when the real struggle begins, nor is it by any means those who are most demonstrative in the early part of the fight who acquit themselves best in it. History tells us that men and officers who have thought most seriously of the duty to be performed and the perils run in battle, are those who have ever acquitted themselves best. This was the case in the armies of William the Conqueror as compared with those of Harold, in those of Cromwell as compared with the Cavaliers, and in the late war, in those of the Prussians, as compared with those of the French.

A man should bear in mind that his great object is to economise his strength in battle. Men fatigued, must necessarily be beaten by those who are fresh. Besides this, when a battle begins no man can say when or how operations are to end, or what amount of exertion he may have to perform. Hence, again, the necessity of having strength to begin with. There will be use for all a man has before many hours are over. It is always desirable that a soldier should not enter battle after a fast, that he should have in his havresac a small reserve of food to use when necessary. The man who is under the influence of drink, if he does not commit an indiscretion and get wounded, soon lags behind, and is worse than useless.

BEARDS.—There is much said about the wearing of beards by soldiers, and the restrictions under which they are in this respect, as compared with sailors and policemen. On active service, and on some foreign stations, beards are permitted, but not so in the United Kingdom. They have been advocated on the score of health; but considering the youth of the great majority of soldiers of the present day, and how few could sport good beards even were they permitted to do so, it cannot be said that much force applies to this reason. The one argument in their favour is that shaving takes up -time, and is more or less a trouble.

BEDDING.—Irrespective of the periods laid down in " orders " for changing the different articles of bedding, the soldier should know that cleanliness in this respect is essential to his health. Whenever, therefore, the sheets or blankets become accidentally soiled, they should be changed. The practice of getting out of bed and going outside at night, without clothes or shoes on, renders the soldier very liable to a chill, and subsequent attack of illness more or less severe. So, also, the practice of throwing himself half undressed on his bed when hot, or leaving his clothes off at night, as men often do in India, is often followed by serious illness. The oftener it is possible to expose bedding in which men sleep to the sun and breeze, the better it is for purposes of health.

BEDS IN BARRACKS.—The "regulation" bedstead is 6 feet 4 inches in length, by 2 feet 3 inches in breadth. It is calculated that in barracks the interval between adjoining bedsteads should be a foot and a half, that between the foot of *opposite* row 6 feet at least, although there are many circumstances under which neither is attainable. Beds should be at least 6 inches from the wall, their feet directed to the centre of the room, and whenever it can be avoided, they should not be placed in corners or recesses, where free circulation of air is impossible. Everything over a foot and a half between adjoining beds is so much gained for health ; everything under is so much lost. In *hospital* the rule generally observed is that the spaces between beds shall be equal to the breadth of a bedstead —that is, 2 feet 3 inches.

BEER.—In reality the use of beer to excess is little if at all less injurious to health than that of spirits. In small quantities taken after the heat of the day is over, say a pint, its injurious effects are at their minimum ; but taken in large quantities, or during hot weather, it stupefies the person, incapacitates him for work, and renders him liable to illness, either fulluess in the head, or *oppression* in the chest. When long indulged in it deranges digestion, renders the stomach irritable, induces a feeling of sickness and want of appetite for meals, and, moreover, tends to cause diseases of the liver and kidneys. In India and other hot countries the free use of beer, especially during the day-time, often leads to fatal attacks of *heat apoplexy*. Good beer should be clear and free from sediment when left standing, with moderate degree of white froth ; have a pleasant bitter taste, neither too bitter nor *clammy*. What is called old ale is only beer that has become a little acid, and the use of such is liable to induce diarrhœa and pains in the stomach. It is also wise to warn soldiers against *doctored* beer, such as they sometimes get in low public houses. There is reason to believe that this is often given to them so that they may become *drugged*, and thus the men readily fall into the power of loose women attached to the houses, or perhaps get robbed.

BELTS OF FLANNEL are issued as part of the soldier's kit, but it is well to impress upon him their great value for preserving health. Their use often prevents cholera, colic, or dysentery, as their neglect induces those diseases. In damp and unhealthy countries, on the march, and in bivouac they are extremely useful, and should never be dispensed with during the night, at which time the liability to such diseases is greatest.—*See* CUMMUR-BUNDS.

BILLETS.—Unfortunately it so happens that the owners of public-houses in which soldiers are billeted sometimes endeavour to make them spend money in drink. There

B

are also various other temptations thrown in their way,
including loose women whom they meet in the town ; and
the man who values his own comfort and health will avoid
both.   There is no doubt that infectious diseases are
sometimes contracted in billets, notwithstanding that the
officers take care to make all preliminary inquiries.   All
that a soldier can do is to look carefully about, and if he
finds anything wrong, tell his sergeant, who will report it
to his officer.   He should be careful to see that his bed is
clean.—*See* SPACE.

BISCUIT.—This form of *bread* should, as a rule, be soaked
either in soup, tea, or coffee, before being eaten.   If used
in a dry state it acts as a sponge in the stomach, soaks up
the natural juices, and in the long run deranges digestion.
The French soldiers are very particular on this point.
They say that its continued use causes obstinate diarrhœa ;
and certainly it does heartburn.   It is only issued when
fresh bread is unobtainable.

BITES are sometimes caused by men, sometimes by
animals.   If by a dog, they are sometimes followed by
hydrophobia, a mortal disease ; and the fact should be
borne in mind that an animal of this kind if enraged, may
produce the disease.   Hence soldiers should avoid going
near dogs while fighting.   In the cavalry and artillery
bites are occasionally caused by horses.   In cases of such
injuries the best thing to be done until the person can be
seen by a surgeon is to bathe the wound instantly with
warm or hot water, so as to encourage the bleeding from
them.
    In BITES OF TARANTULAS, CENTIPEDES, &c., apply the
oily matter in a tobacco pipe, spirits, hartshorn, ipecacu-
anha, honey, or sugar.—*See* SNAKE BITE.
    It is recommended in the case of bite by an enraged
or rabid dog, to place without delay a ligature or bandage
upon the wounded limb at a point nearer to the body,
provided it be possible to do so.   The wound itself should

be pressed strongly with a view to thus cause the exit of the poisonous matter. The wounded part should then be placed in warm water, and the services of a surgeon obtained without delay.

BIVOUAC.—It is comparatively seldom, now-a-days, that our soldiers are called upon to bivouac. It may be possible that some day or other it will again be required of them. If it be so in a hot country, their first duty should be to see that the ground is clear of noxious creatures, such as snakes, scorpions, and centipedes. If circumstances permit a man to get behind an undulation, and so guard against the wind, he will of course do so. Wherever practicable the boots should be taken off, and the feet covered in the blanket carried by the man. The face and ears should be covered at night. Officers will, of course, avoid bivouacking upon ground that had shortly before been similarly used. In looking out for a place to bivouac singly, bear in mind that a wall or other screen, 18 inches high, is sufficient to protect a man from the strength of a storm. Trees are delusive ; they act as a shade, but not as a shelter; they rather make eddies of wind, rendering their presence objectionable on the ground for bivouac. Hillocks and undulations of the ground should be taken advantage of. Low-lying ground should, however, be avoided, and that slightly elevated selected. Avoid also the near neighbourhood of water, if possible, in whatever climate. In some cases—as in the sandy plains of Africa, India, and Australia—a man may make himself tolerably comfortable by " burying " himself pretty deeply in the surface sand at night, leaving his head clear. If a fire or embers of a camp-fire are obtainable, a man may, by bivouacking close to them, make himself tolerably comfortable. In all cases the body should have sufficient covering above, as well as below, if that be possible. In the retreat from Moscow, many a soldier saved his own life by bivouacking under the lee of a dead horse. If a man has not sufficient clothing to keep him warm in the bivouac, his sufferings at night are often fearful. He should also remember that some protection between him and the ground is as necessary, or perhaps more so, than clothing over him, and make use of grass, twigs, and shrubs as a kind of mattress under him. A temporary shelter may be made by driving into the ground forked sticks four feet long, placing a pole between them, and resting branches against them on the windward side. When military considerations permit, fires should be lighted in circular clusters, and the men lie down between them. They should then lie in squads, spreading one or two blankets on the ground, or over straw if obtainable, the remaining blankets being spread over them. In wet or cold weather hot coffee should be issued to the men before they lie down to sleep, and not more than one-half of their numbers should do so at the same time. The application of oil or grease to the hands and face is a good protection against the effects of cold in bivouac.

BLISTERS ON THE FEET.—The best method of treating blisters on the feet is, if they have not broken, to run a fine needle and thread through them, so that the contents may be discharged, and then the skin will adhere to the raw surface underneath and so protect it. Those that have broken should be treated with a little suet or simple ointment on a piece of cloth, after the feet have been well bathed in warm water and dried. On starting afterwards on the march, the soldier should be careful that his sock is without holes in it, that it is properly put on his bad foot, and that the boot is soft. After a few days' march we hear no more of blistered feet.—*See* FEET. Another application to blistered feet consists of a mixture of spirits and melted tallow. This, if put on at night, is said to cure the blisters. To prevent them, apply soap to the inside of the sock, so as to make a lather, before starting on the march. A raw egg broken into the boot before putting it on very greatly softens the leather. A good plan also is after a march to change the socks, right to left and left to right, or turn them.

BLOOD, SPITTING OF.—This comes on with cough more or less severe, the expectoration or spittle being at first streaked with blood, but afterwards the blood following the cough in greater or smaller quantities, according to the severity of the attack. There is a feeling of oppression upon the chest. After each fit of coughing the blood is frothy and of a light red colour. The person has a feeling as if the desire to cough were situated deep in the chest. Breathing becomes difficult; there is a feeling of heat and tickling in the throat. This kind of illness must always be considered as very serious to the patient, it being in many cases the forerunner of incurable disease. The first thing to be done is to open the clothes of the man; lay him flat, bathe the chest with cold water, and if there be any vinegar in the barrack-room, to give him a little mixed with water. He should *be carried* to hospital; not made to walk.

BOOTS.—Much of the power of marching of a man depends upon the manner in which his boots are fitted. Too large a boot *frays* and injures the foot; too small a boot destroys it, and lays up the man. Certain allowance should be made, when trying on a boot, for the expanse of the foot in length and breadth while walking, and this is greater in a fleshy than a hard bony foot. For the purpose of real work the boots should be well greased, as well to render them waterproof as to keep them flexible. They should be well cleaned inside, if necessary. Should be so made as to fit tight—but not too tight—just in front of the instep, be broad in the heels, and at the toes.

BRUISES may be of any degree of severity, from what merely causes slight discolouration of the skin to that which destroys all feeling in the part. Such as are usually met with may be caused by blows, falls, kicks, &c. A very common seat of them is the parts around the eyes. The best immediate application is cold water, or water containing some spirits or vinegar. A thin piece of cloth should be soaked in either, and applied. Cold will be produced by evaporation of the lotion, and this will check in some manner the effusion of blood. Severe bruises of the chest or belly may cause death by injury to the parts contained in these cavities respectively. A favourite application to those in the limbs or face is tincture of arnica; but spirits in any other form would be just as good.

BURNS AND SCALDS.—These injuries may be of all degrees of severity, from slight redness of the skin to complete destruction of the vitality of the injured part. Those indicated here, however, are the comparatively slight ones, such as occur by accidents about barracks; injuries of this kind, such as happen in battle by the explosion of mines, tumbrils, &c., being usually far more urgent in their nature. If a man has accidentally got burnt or scalded, let the injured part be freed from clothing as quickly as possible. If cold water is obtainable, throw some upon the part; or, in the case of a limb, let it be placed in a vessel full of it. If the surface is only reddened, or slightly blistered, this may be sufficient for the time being, or, if not, the part may be gently smeared with oil or grease, or dusted with flower. In the more severe cases, when the skin is swept clean off, the best kind of first dressing is carded cotton soaked in oil, or white of egg, or whitewash.

CAMP.—The straw or other material used for bedding in a standing camp should be changed as often as possible, irrespective of the *Regulations* upon the subject. Cleanliness within and without the tents should be carefully maintained; the committal of nuisance around them checked by the soldiers themselves. The slaughter yard and latrines should be as far as possible from the camp, and soldiers will understand the necessity of the whole force changing ground occasionally, and avoiding sites of previous camps. In some countries it is dangerous when pitching a camp to take off the surface of the ground, disease being often produced in this way. Hence it must be done cautiously, if at all. Men should avoid rushing out of the tents at night half naked to go to the latrines. A chill thus produced may give rise to serious disease, dysentery more especially. They should be careful when encamped to have plenty of warm clothing; while asleep, to wear their flannel binders at night. They should take every opportunity of washing their linen. Whenever they can do so they will find it very refreshing to take their boots off before going to bed. For the sake of dividing work, the plan followed in the French Army is that 14 privates and 1 non-commissioned officer usually are told off to a tent. The privates are divided thus :—6 tent men, 2 water men, 1 cook, 3 for duty if required. Each man thus soon learns what he has to do, and should do it. On arriving in camp, if the men are hot they should not take off their coats too soon; when the tents are pitched, then is the time for them to change their underclothing, dry and brush what has been worn, and make their own ablutions. The maintenance of cleanliness in camp is necessary for the well-being of all. Hence, all good officers are very strict in regard to this matter, and soldiers should for their own sakes be equally particular.

CAMP REQUISITES FOR OFFICERS.—The following is a list of articles to be taken as equipment by officers going on service, or to the *Manœuvres*, now becoming a regular part of military training. The list is taken partly from Sir G. Worlesley's Soldiers' Pocket-book, partly from lists of outfitters, viz.: *To be worn on the person*— Shako, tunic, trousers, shooting boots, socks (woollen), drawers, flannel shirt, silk pocket handkerchief, gaiters, clasp-knife, drinking-cup and water-bottle, telescope and compass attached to it, watch, waterproof coat and havresac.

To be carried in the valise, according to Horse Guards' pattern, itself forming a bed :—1 great coat, 1 blanket, 1 pair of trousers, 1 pair shooting boots, 6 pairs boot laces, 2 pairs of worsted socks, 1 pair drawers, 1 flannel shirt, 1 silk pocket handkerchief, 1 woollen nightcap, 1 holdall—containing 1 comb, 1 hair-brush, 1 tooth-brush, 1 pair scissors, 1 soap box, 1 small sponge, 1 clothes'-brush, 1 housewife, 1 tin of dubbing, 1 portfolio, with pen, ink, and paper, 1 journal-book, 1 cholera belt, 1 calico bandage, 1 candle lamp and candles (these are put up together by out-fitters), 1 tin match-box, 2 tin plates, 1 cup in leather bag, containing knife, fork, spoon, pepper and salt pots, a map of the country, and an india-rubber basin. These and the valise weigh about 40 lbs.

As furniture, he should have 1 bedstead, 12 lbs.; air pillow, ½ lb.; bath and sponge bag, 2 lbs.; wash-hand stand, 2 lbs.; bucket, 9 ozs.; camp stool, 8 ozs.; lantern and box of candles, 1 to 4 lbs., unless these be in the valise kit. Total, 29 lbs. 14 ozs., according to the list printed at Aldershot.

Canteen for cooking, if each officer carries his own knife, fork, and spoon,—1 camp kettle, cover and strap, tripod, boiling-pot and cover, stew-pan and cover, sugar canister, tea, coffee, butter, tin canister containing pepper box, mus-tard pot, and salt cellar; 2 saucepans, frypan, gridiron cook's knife, fork, and iron spoon, tea kettle. All these weigh 17 lbs. 7 oz.; fit one within the other, and are secured by a strap around the whole.

The following is a list of clothing used by the men of the *Red River Expedition,* viz. :—*On the person*—1 flannel shirt, 1 pair woollen socks, 1 pair buff moccasins, 1 forage cap, peak and cover, 1 serge frock with pockets, 1 pair serge trousers, 1 havresac, 1 clasp knife, 1 tin cup, 1 waist belt, 1 mess tin, 1 great coat (both these in the pack). *In the pack,*—1 flannel shirt, 2 pairs woollen socks, 1 pair ammu-nition boots, 1 thick woollen night cap, 1 towel, 1 piece of soap, 1 brush (clothes or boot), 1 comb, 1 linen bandage, 1 small book, 1 housewife, knife, fork, and spoon.

CAMPAIGNING, *see* SERVICE.

CATARRH OR COMMON COLD.—Men who are exposed to vicissitudes of weather and season, as soldiers necessarily are, suffer considerably from these affections. As precau-tions, they should wear plenty of warm clothing, avoid remaining in wet garments if possible, and endeavour to go on duty undebilitated by debauch. If attacked with *a cold*, let the subject of it take plenty of hot drinks, place his feet in warm water, and go to bed, unless he has it in his power to proceed direct to hospital. Catarrh, if neglected, is apt to end in one or other of the severe affections of the chest, as bronchitis or pneumonia, either of which is difficult to be got rid of, and may endanger life. As to "working off" a cold, this is only possible when the attack is a slight one.

CARRYING A SICK OR WOUNDED COMRADE.—*Stretchers* are usually provided in every regiment for the purpose. In laying a sick or injured man upon one, care should be taken that he is placed in a position or attitude to give him the greatest measure of comfort under the circumstances. As a rule he is best placed upon his back, his limbs stretched out straight, unless actually displaced by the wound or accident; but there should always be a pillow under his head, and his neck and chest should be left free by the coat being unbuttoned. In cases of accident or sudden illness, the great mistake made by soldiers is to be too hurried; another, in being *too rough*. The person should be laid gently upon the stretcher; his head, arms, and feet all supported upon it, instead of dangling from it; one man at either end should then raise it gently, the one at the *foot* end with his *back* to the patient, and then should move off slowly with *a broken* step, so as to avoid shaking the sufferer. A comrade at either side may, with one hand, support the middle of each pole of the stretcher.—*See Stretchers.*

CHAFING.—Some men suffer from chafing between the thighs when on the march, and others from what is commonly known as *losing leather* from riding. Good-fitting drawers, of cotton or other soft material, are good preservatives against such accidents. When they do occur, the parts should be moistened with oil or grease, kept thoroughly clean, and after the march is over, and ablutions performed, dusted with flour, starch, or other absorbent powder.

CHAPPED HANDS OR FACE.—This is one of the common effects of cold. It is always more or less disagreeable ; but in the case of the hands particularly so, bleeding often taking place from cracks in the skin over the points. It may or may not be attended by chilblains. Generally, however, it is so. The best preventatives consist of spirits and oil freely rubbed in morning and evening, gloves, especially leather gloves, being worn throughout the day. A thin leather glove underneath, with woollen or other gloves outside, form the best preservative of warmth for the hand, and consequent preventative of *chaps*.

CHARCOAL.—There is danger of a man being poisoned by the vapours of burning charcoal if he permits himself to go to sleep in a room where a vessel containing this kind of fuel is *alight*. To avoid this accident it is necessary that the flame should have entirely ceased before the person settles down to rest ; at the same time it is necessary to remember that the quantity of *carbonic acid,* or the poisonous gas given out, is less when the flame is bright than when it is beginning to burn or is nearly extinguished. To recover a person from the effects of this gas, let him be exposed to the fresh air, bathe the head and face with water or water and vinegar. If he is unconscious; lay him upon the ground, raise his head, sponge his face and chest with vinegar and water, rub the arms and legs, apply hartshorn fumes to the nostrils, or tickle them and the mouth with a feather. When recovery begins, place him in a warm bed, and give a little stimulant.—*See* COAL.

CHEESE.—This for the soldier is both agreeable to the taste and useful as a supplementary article of diet, and, as a rule, forms, with biscuit or bread, a favourite " snack " at the regimental canteen. On the march it is always advisable, whenever there is a probability of delay in the issue of regular rations, to have a small piece of cheese. This is partly provided for by *Regulations ;* but soldiers would do well to look after themselves in this as in a good many other respects.

CHILBLAINS.—These take place at the beginning of winter, usually on parts that had previously suffered from cold. They occur in the form of painful and inflamed tumours of greater or less extent upon the hands, feet, or ears, and are, in reality, but mild forms of *frost-bite.* When they begin to take place, and before being "broken," apply a little camphor and oil to them, wear very warm socks and gloves, and use active exercise. When chilblains are severe, or have formed ulcers, the soldier should consult his medical officer. These affections, although generally without any particular danger, ought by no means to be neglected, as they sometimes degenerate into painful and obstinate ulcers.

CHOKING.—If a foreign substance, as a piece of meat, &c., be retained in the throat, proceed thus :—Strike the back, endeavour to provoke sneezing, try to provoke vomiting by introducing into the throat a feather smeared in oil. If a bone be the object stuck, endeavour to get it swallowed, as by giving a morsel of bread-crumb or drinking a quantity of water. Another plan is to extend the tongue, place upon it a piece of tobacco or other irritating substance, so that by causing motion in it and inducing an attempt at vomiting the foreign body may sometimes be dislodged and thrown out. By poking the finger into the throat, unless care be taken, more harm than good is likely to be done. The man should be taken to hospital without delay.

CHOLERA (*see also* EPIDEMICS).—When this scourge is anticipated, and during its prevalence, the best exertions of the higher authorities, as well as of the regimental officers, are directed to its aversion, if possible, or, at all events, to its mitigation. Many of the measures taken are in their nature beyond the means of the generality of soldiers to comprehend fully; but others are quite within their knowledge, and, in fact, their success depends in a great measure upon the co-operation and good sense of the men themselves. They can understand that by change of locality, by good ventilation, the separation of patients attacked from others in hospital, and the breaking-up of regiments into various portions, all being sent away in different directions, all that is possible is thus done to prevent the spread of this disease, one of the peculiarities of which is that it clings to masses of people crowded together, whether they be so in camps, barracks, or cities. They can also readily understand how necessary it is to avoid panic, to refrain from excesses which, in reality, increase liability to attack, and diminish the chances of recovery of those attacked; also that they should wear their flannel belts, be on the alert to take, if attacked with diarrhœa, some of the medicine which, under such circumstances, the surgeon has 'sent to the non-commissioned officers for distribution, as well as how necessary it is that they should be taken to hospital at the very earliest possible moment after the seizure. The most frequent time for attack is towards morning.

Cleanliness is absolutely indispensable to health, whether of the individual or the mass. It is, if possible. even more so on the march and bivouac than in barracks. Under all circumstances the hands, face, neck, and upper part of the chest should be washed with cold water, the teeth brushed with a hard brush, the hair combed and brushed. Cleanliness of the mouth cannot be too much insisted upon, not only for the comfort of the man himself, but for that of his comrades right and left of him. This precaution is by no means attended to as it should be; but considering what an offensive and injurious thing a foul breath is, surely the propriety of averting it as far as possible is self-evident. The feet should be carefully washed as often as possible. On the march or active service this is, if possible, more necessary than in quarters. The nails of the fingers and toes should be trimmed once a week, those of the latter, especially of the great toes, being cut *square*, by which means in-growing of the corner into the flesh may best be guarded against.

But although under ordinary circumstances absolute cleanliness is necessary for health, and will be insisted upon by the responsible officers, there are conditions connected with military service where limitations must exist in this respect, as, for example, in very cold climates and in very inclement weather. In a temperate climate cleanliness must be insisted upon. In barracks the air becomes foul to a fearful degree if this is neglected; the mass of men become unhealthy, and diseases such as arise from *over-crowding* occur. Cleanliness of his person, cleanliness as regards his surroundings, must be looked upon as consti-tuting, in ordinary times, the great safeguards of the health of the soldier.

CLIMATE.—The soldier must be prepared to serve in all climates,—those that are extreme, those that are hot, cold, dry, or damp. It is not to be denied that " climate " exerts a very great influence upon the health and constitution. Animals and plants transported to climates different from that of their own native country suffer in quite an equal extent to what man does. No doubt man has it in his power by suitable arrangements to modify, to a certain extent, the effects of climate ; but on the other hand, by neglecting those arrangements, and what is still worse, by running into excesses and indiscretions such as would have a pernicious influence even in his own country, he increases the risks of injury to health, and perhaps death, to which he is exposed. Whether a man may after a time become *accustomed* to particular climates is another matter ; but unless care, with moderation and temperance, be observed, life will certainly not be sufficiently prolonged to give the *experiment* a fair chance of succeeding.

When a soldier arrives for the first time in a hot climate he should be careful to regulate his conduct. He should expose himself as little as possible, be moderate as regards food and drink, avoid exciting drinks in considerable quantity, be careful in the use of native fruits, wear loosely-made clothes, and, if the atmosphere be moist, use such as are made of woollen material. Abundant sleep is desirable, and bathing should be regularly practised.

CLOTHING.—The dress of the soldier is determined by *regulation.* Nevertheless, it is well known that during autumn and winter, in mountainous countries and on the line of march, it is right to dress in woollen clothes, whatever be the state of or kind of weather, on account of the changes that may occur in it. This rule is also more or less applicable to hot countries or those of extreme climates, such as some parts of India and China. In these the body clothes best suited for all purposes are those that consist of thin woollen material. During great heat cotton trousers are perhaps most suitable. The French troops in Algeria find cotton or linen trousers agreeable, as our own do in hot countries. Clothes should be changed whenever they become wet. This precaution is absolutely essential, in order to avoid evil results. An immensity of evil is done by having the collar of the tunic too tight; this impedes the circulation of the blood, and becomes a source of disease of the heart. So also, the trousers, if too tight round the waist, interfere with the soldier in his drill, especially when kneeling, and suddenly getting up again, sometimes giving rise to *rupture.* Woollen articles of clothing should be often exposed to the air, and beaten, so as to free them from dust; the trousers and tunics turned inside out, especially after a march or drill, when they are perhaps tainted with perspiration. When ordered on service, the articles of clothing of all kinds should be new, or as nearly new as the man can manage to have them. This the officers will doubtless see to.—*See* DRAWERS.

Soldiers should guard against insufficient clothing in

cold or wet climates ; nor should they be in a hurry to
leave off those worn in winter on the approach of summer.
They can always make use of old tunics to make them into
vests for winter wear.   The older the soldier, or the more
he has suffered from illness, especially abroad, the greater
care he requires to pay to his clothing, that it be warm
and commodious. The young and robust need less clothing
than the older and more feeble ; nevertheless, they require
much more care in this respect than they often take ;
but, under all circumstances, that worn should be sufficient
to prevent the person from suffering from rapid and great
changes of weather or season.

To Dry Wet Clothes on Service.—Make a dome-
shaped framework of twigs by bending each twig inward
into a half circle, and planting both ends of it in the
ground.   A smouldering fire having been made inside this
dome, lay the clothes over the framework.   This is convenient, if other means than wind and sun are needed, but
usually all that is required is to hang the clothes upon
trees or shrubs, where they may be freely exposed to the
breeze.   This plan is generally followed by travellers and
explorers, and may easily be adopted by soldiers in the
field.

Coal, Vapour of.—The vapour of a coal fire when
left in a room where men sleep is only less dangerous to
life than that from charcoal, because the gases mixed in it,
including sulphurous acid, sulphuretted and carburetted
hydrogen, are of themselves so irritating as to give warning
of their presence by causing sneezing.   Nevertheless, if
actual loss of life does not occur from the presence of coal
vapour in rooms, headache, feverishness, and other unpleasant results arise, to guard against which all that is
required is to see that fires are completely extinguished in
the rooms before you go to bed.   To recover from the
effects of vapour of this kind, take a walk in the open air,
bathe the head and body in *cold* water.—*See* Charcoal.

COLD.—If a soldier is found *benumbed* from cold, remove him to an unheated room; open the windows; rub the body and limbs with cold water; practice artificial respiration as in cases of *drowning;* then place him in a bed, and when he begins to revive give him a little warm tea. The application of hot bottles to the person should be avoided; nor should a fire be lighted in the room. In order to protect the body against the cold of the weather, the evident plan is to use plenty of woollen clothing, including stockings. A plan recommended in France is to have two cotton shirts, one over the other, flannel being still worn next the skin.—*See also* CATARRH.

COLIC.—Severe twisting pain in the belly without diarrhœa. Apply cloths wrung out of hot water to the stomach, taking care that they are not so hot as to blister. Give hot drinks, with any aromatic, as cinnamon, &c., that is readily available, while arrangements are being made to send the man affected to hospital. The affection is usually caused by having the feet wet and neglecting to change the socks, or by exposure to a current of damp or cold wind with the *stomach* insufficiently clothed.

CONDUCT.—A man's personal conduct has very great influence upon his own health, for good or for bad, and often affects that of his comrades also. Thus, he who leads a regular and temperate life, avoiding public-houses, brothels, and other places where vice and disease are usually met with, is surely more likely to be unaffected by either than the reckless or thoughtless man who frequents both, and indulges in their so-called "pleasures." A soldier should remember that as such, *discipline* requires that he exert command over himself, and this accordingly he must learn to do. If respectful to his superiors and yielding willing obedience, he will be kindly treated by all, whereas if disrespectful and obstinate he will find his life by no means a happy one. Every soldier should, as soon as possible, make himself acquainted with the *orders* and *regulations* according to which he is now to be treated, and learn to accommodate himself to them.

CONVALESCENCE.—Medical officers prescribe the regimen to be followed during convalescence from illness ; nevertheless there are some points that are altogether influenced by the soldier himself, and it is well that his attention should be directed to them. It is essential that instructions given by the surgeon be rigidly followed. It will be well for a man to consider what have been the causes of his illness, and thus learn how for the future they are to be best avoided. Probably, there will be few who may not find something to correct or avoid in their manner of life, their food, drink, regulation of their desires and passions, and so on.

COOKING.—Whether it is or is not necessary in India and some other countries similarly situated in this respect that soldiers should all have a practical knowledge of the art of cooking, it is essential for the requirements of war against an enemy in Europe that each should be able to manage for himself. This was demonstrated over and over again during the Franco-German war. The mess-tin may always be used for this purpose, and on service, the readiest and perhaps the best plan of preparing food is to stew the meat with such vegetables as are issued, and with a little seasoning, which can generally be obtained. If time does not admit of this, the meat may be broiled, and to do this the French troops in Algeria used to make temporary gridirons of their ramrods, but the latter being now abolished, men must obtain what other means they can. The French believe that meat is more wholesome when stewed or cooked as broth than when roasted. They consider that the use of roasted or broiled meat on the march or on service causes dysentery and other diseases of the bowels, as happened during the expedition to Russia in 1812.

See Queen's Regulations, on the subject of COOKING.

The process of cooking meat ought always to be complete. Underdone meat is to many persons offensive and indigestible, and its use renders all liable to become affected by TAPE-WORM, the germs of which are in such a case not deprived of their vitality. Certain kinds of sausages and meat, unless well cooked, are liable to cause disease of a severe nature. In fact, no kind of *meat* ought to be eaten in an uncooked state.

CORNS ON THE FEET are, for the most part, caused by wearing too tight or too hard boots. There are persons, however, who are subject to them whether their boots be large or small, and are rendered thereby hardly able to march. The corns may take place upon the more prominent parts of the foot, or between the toes; in the latter, as *soft* corns. To relieve them as much as possible, bathe the feet well in warm water, then with a sharp knife cut off as much as can safely be done. For the soft ones, apply some carded cotton soaked in oil. A good plan is, after they are cut and the surface is still moist, to rub the surface gently with *caustic* (nitrate of silver) taking care that this is not done to too great an extent, as, in that case, the parts will become blistered. A thin crust will form on the surface, and by repeating the application every three days or so, not only will the pain be rendered less, but will be easy to take off the crust by means of the nail, and with it, often the " *core.*"

COUGH.—The fact of a man suffering from cough for some time indicates the existence of mischief in the windpipe or chest, for the removal of which medical treatment is absolutely necessary. Cough in the early morning, especially if attended by expectoration of pellet-like masses of matter, indicates liability to consumption, if not, indeed, the beginning of that disease. If the *pellets* expectorated are streaked with blood, the symptom is always of a serious nature. Under no circumstances should the existence of cough be neglected. Even when it is habitual, or confined to the winter season, it requires to be attended to and treated. Unless it be so, it will sooner or later end in serious danger to the sufferer.

CROWDING.—The regulations of the service make very definite arrangements so as to prevent too great a number of men being placed together in the same barrack-room. It is, nevertheless, well that the soldiers should themselves know that to the practice of overcrowding, such as it used to prevail, was due the fearful extent to which *typhus* fever raged in our army, and that to the modern and improved arrangements in this and other respects we can attribute the absolute extinction of that, as well as some other diseases among them. Still, there are evils which are more or less inseparable from the fact of considerable bodies of men occupying the same room, the risks arising from this circumstance being increased by the practice of huddling together, more especially if ventilation and personal cleanliness be neglected. Of these evils, pulmonary consumption is a principal; headaches, sickness, faintness, and loss of strength, are among the other effects. The men should, therefore, avoid bringing their bedsteads nearer each other than the regulated distance between them, namely, a foot and a half to two feet in barracks, and one and a half in huts. They should also remember that although the *cubic* measurements be sufficient according to official measurement, yet unless the superficial space be also good, injury to the health of individuals will be the result. Another point to bear in mind is, that wherever persons are crowded together, there, epidemics when they occur prevail with greatest intensity.

CUMMURBUNDS.—*See* BELTS.—These have been found of the greatest service by the French in Algeria and by our troops in India during the Sepoy mutiny. They protect the loins against the effects of the sun, and guard the stomach against chills. The long kind of cloth such as that made for the purpose is best suited for it. The *cummurbund* to be worn during the day, the flannel belt at

night. On home service, and in temperate climates generally, the regulations in force prevent the wearing of anything in the shape of a *cummurbund* outside the uniform;
on actual service, however, these regulations no doubt
would be relaxed, and whenever they are so, soldiers will
derive the greatest advantage from adopting the precaution of thus protecting the loins and "stomach."

CUTS.—*See* WOUNDS BY SWORDS.—In cases of accidental
cuts, such as soldiers meet with in barracks, the first thing
to be done is to press the cut surfaces together to prevent
the bleeding that would otherwise take place. In the
case of a hand or superficial wound in a limb, this may be
all that is needed. In such a case a few turns of a bandage rolled round the part may be all that is required.
The cloth gets soaked with the oozing blood, then dry so
as to form a crust, and thus prevents access of air to the
wound, which will heal rapidly. If the wound is of a
more serious nature so as to open a blood-vessel, the flow
of blood will speedily indicate its actual nature. The
shortest way in such a case is for a comrade to grasp the
part as tightly as he can, and maintain his hold until the
arrival of a surgeon.

DEATH.—Under ordinary circumstances the proportion
of men per regiment who die naturally is tolerably constant. It varies, however, according to conditions and
station, and is altogether placed beyond regular calculation
by the occurrence of *Epidemics.* As a rule, the death-rate
from all causes amounts to about 20 per 1,000 annually of
the troops on home service; on foreign stations it is considerably more, besides the numbers who every year become unfit for service, and are *invalided,* Soldiers should
study these matters, as so much depends upon themselves
as regards the diminution of the death-rates in regiments.

DIARRHŒA.—Use hot drinks whether of gruel, tea, or
rice water; keep the stomach and feet warm. Hot soup is

very grateful until the sufferer can be taken to hospital. If a little ginger, cinnamon, or oil of peppermint, a small pinch or a few drops should be added to the hot drink. The French are fond of using a weak infusion of camomile against diarrhœa, and often cultivate the plant for the purpose. It does not grow, however, in many places to which British soldiers are sent, but there are always bitter and aromatic plants such as are used by the natives of different countries, and the employment of which often keep off this as well as other diseases. The application to the stomach of a hot brick rolled up in a blanket or other woollen cloth is beneficial as well as grateful. Perfect rest should be observed, and unless the person attacked can be taken to hospital or otherwise prescribed for, he ought to remain in bed.

DIGESTION.—The process of digestion proceeds best when a man has it in his power to remain at rest for some time after a meal, or at most if the exercise be moderate, as in walking. In fact, a man is incapable of very violent exercise while digestion is going on, fullness of the head and sickness being often caused by it. Exercise and an active life, however, if taken at suitable times, and then rest immediately after meals, increase both the appetite and power of digestion. The time required for the complete digestion of various kinds of food depends upon their nature. For soldiers it will be sufficient to know that beef and mutton require three to four hours, salt beef four and a half, potatoes and bread about three.

DISEASE.—*See also* SICKNESS.—*Concealment* of disease is a military offence and insures liability to punishment. Irrespective of that, however, the soldier should bear in mind that disease in a general sense is most readily curable in the early stages, and that in some cases, if once it obtains full possession of the system, its effects never can be got rid of, but slowly and painfully drag him down to death. This is especially the case with the class well known to soldiers as "*the disease.*" Sores upon the body, disfigurement, painful affections of the joints and bones, are its immediate results. If ever a man who has once suffered constitutionally from it marries, the chances are that his children will be diseased also. Hence surely he ought, when unfortunate enough to become affected, to take the very earliest opportunity of consulting the surgeon instead of *quacking*, or altogether neglecting himself, as is often done, until the mischief now indicated has taken place, There are certain *diseases* incidental to *Service*, such as typhus fever, dysentery, cholera, scurvy, &c., against all of which the medical officers take steps for protecting the men; yet unless the soldiers themselves are careful, the efforts of others will more or less fail. In campaigns it often happens that the deaths by disease are as 7 or 8 to one, as compared with the losses in battle and by wounds. Hence the necessity of men guarding against illness is evident.

DISINFECTANTS.—As a rule it may be said of disinfectants that their use would be unnecessary were perfect cleanliness observed. In some instances they become necessary as a temporary means of destroying emanations that might otherwise prove injurious, and which arise in consequence of defects in drains, &c. Soldiers should know, however, that where disinfectants are needed cleanliness has not been attended to as it ought to have been, and that probably the fault rests with themselves or their predecessors in the same barracks. The *disinfectants* allowed by Regulation are *lime* and *carbolic acid.* The former is often ineffectual, and when used for latrines and urinals, after a time renders matters worse than they were before; the latter is only useful for destroying "organic" matters, not for *inorganic*, as sulphuretted hydrogen and ammonia arising from sewers and latrines. For *disinfecting* purposes chlorine gas and carbolic acid are those best adapted. The former is produced by pouring a little sulphuric acid upon common table salt in a saucer.

DISLOCATIONS.—These imply the unnatural separation or displacement of the bones forming a joint. They are usually caused by a blow or fall, and can be at once recognised by the fact of the joint affected being thrown out of its natural shape, and being more or less completely immovable. The nature of the accident is recognised by the existence of pain, difficulty of moving the part, deformity, displacement or change of direction of the bones, lengthening or shortening of the joint. Sometimes there is so much swelling as to render it difficult for a surgeon to detect the actual nature of the injury. All that can be done is to place the limb in the most comfortable position possible until the sufferer is carried to hospital, supporting the part if need be by pillows, or by the hands of comrades.—*See* FRACTURES.

DRAGOONS, WEIGHT OF.—The average net weight of a dragoon is about 11½ stone, of a lancer 11 stone, of a hussar 10 stone, 3 lbs. That of their dress, arms, accoutrements, ammunition, and equipment worn on the person, is respectively about 31 lbs. 6 oz., 32 lbs. 4 oz., and 31 lbs. 14 oz. Adding the weight of the water-bottle full, 2 lbs. 4 oz., and 2 days' rations for the man, 4 lbs., the total weight carried by the horses of our cavalry is—Heavies, 19 st. 2 lbs. ; Lancers, 18 st. 10 lbs. ; Hussars, 17 st. 13 lbs. ; to these weights must be added one day's corn for the horse (Wolseley). There are particular kinds of diseases to which a dragoon is more liable than an infantry soldier. Of these, ruptures, swelled testicle, and strains of the muscles of the thigh are the most frequent. To guard against the second named the use of *suspensors* is recommended. It has been said that *hæmorrhoids* are more frequent in the mounted than in the unmounted branches, but statistics do not support this belief.

DRAWERS.—Although not in the list of *necessaries* of a soldier, they not only afford great comfort when worn, but are necessary in order to maintain cleanliness. Rough woollen trowsers, if worn without drawers, not only fret and irritate the limbs and " fork," but soon become offensively dirty, and in consequence unwholesome. In hot countries drawers of *long* cloth are the most comfortable ; in temperate and cold climates those of *wove* cloth or lamb's wool are the best suited for use. Drawers do form part of the kit of the French soldier, and they ought certainly to be used by those of the English army. Soldiers would soon find how greatly they enhance their individual comfort.

DRILLS.—The plan followed in India of giving coffee and biscuit to each man before going to morning drill is absolutely essential to health there, but should be adopted elsewhere when men have to parade before breakfast. Soldiers should know that early drills ensure early hours, and some degree of sobriety the previous night; hence indeed their chief use. Officers do know that the shorter the drill the more attention is paid to it by the men ; the longer and more frequent, the more irksome. It is a necessity of the drills that they involve constrained positions on the part of the soldier. The more speedily the man accommodates himself to what is unavoidable the better it will be in all respects for himself. Some men have a greater aptitude than others in learning this part of their duties. So it is with all other occupations in life. Patience on their own part and that of their teachers, will not only succeed better than hastiness and irritation, but the health of the recruit will thus the better be secured, for many young men *break down* completely in the course of their drill. The periods of the day at which drills should take place depend upon climate and season. In hot countries and seasons early morning is the best time for them ; in cold and winter, the middle of the day.

DRINKS.—Undoubtedly the best *drink* for all purposes is water. It is, however, neither sufficiently pungent or potent for the generality of soldiers ; consequently is seldom used when other descriptions can be got. Effervescing drinks, as soda water, lemonade, ginger beer, &c., are very agreeable, and when properly made, wholesome. So also are *sherbets* of different kinds, as those of lemons, tamarinds, &c., in hot countries. Tea and coffee are excellent. Cold tea the best of all to work upon and undergo fatigue. Wines are little relished by British soldiers, and are moreover expensive; otherwise light kinds are well adapted for hot climates. Unhappily, beer and spirits are the favourite drinks in our army, further remarks regarding both being made under their respective heads.

DROWNING.—Undress, then extend the person upon the ground, laying him slightly upon the right side; raise the head gently; cover the body, if possible, with a warm and dry blanket; apply a hand to each side over the short ribs; gently press, then relax, then press again, and so on, so as to produce a movement of the ribs and chest as nearly as possible like that of natural breathing; the hand of a man being at the same time gently applied to the belly. While this is being done, gently, steadily, and perseveringly, a second man should, if possible, rub with a piece of flannel over the spine of the back. The nostrils should meantime be tickled with a feather. It is useless to pour spirits into the mouth until breathing has become restored. The case should not be given up as hopeless, until pronounced so by the surgeon, who should at once be sent for. It is, of course, necessary in handling the man, to avoid injuring him. Wipe carefully mud and slime from the mouth and nostrils. It may be well at first to place him on his stomach, with the head on a lower level than the body, so that water may be permitted to escape from the mouth; but it is dangerous to the man's life to suspend him with the head directly downwards, as is sometimes recommended by ignorant people.

To Save a Man from Drowning in the Surf—If he is being washed backwards and forwards by the waves his comrades may save him by holding firmly together, each having

hold of the hand of the other, and so forming a line down to
the sea, the nearest one laying hold of the drowning man
as he is washed up to him, and holding him until the
wave recedes, when he is to be drawn on shore before
the next comes in. Strength and steadiness are needed
to do this.

DRUNKENNESS.—It is surely unnecessary to point out to
the soldier that the vice of drunkenness is not only un-
manly in itself, but that it exposes its victim to a great
many causes of injury to health and character. He who
"takes to drink" because he has got into trouble or mis-
fortune, is invariably a *coward*, inasmuch as he prefers to
benumb and destroy his senses rather than face his difficulties like a man. Not only are the greater number of
crimes attended by violence in the army committed as
direct results of drunkenness, but men in this state are
those who mostly meet with accidents, including fractures
and dislocations ; who become the subjects of *contagious*
diseases, and thus are not only rendered unfit for military
duty, but their disability not being attributable to service,
are discharged, it may be with little or no pension, broken
in health, unable to earn their own living, and with only
the alternative of a prison or a poor-house before them.
Literally, and truly, a confirmed drunkard is a worse and
more dangerous animal than are the brute beasts. Every
soldier knows that it is not necessary that a man should
be so many times in an actual state of *intoxication* to constitute himself a drunkard. He who drinks most steadily
is not by any means the one to be oftenest in a state of
actual drunkenness. He is, however, at all times more or
less under its effects; if hurt or sick, has a much worse
chance of recovery than his sober comrades, and sooner or
later gets *delirium tremens,* or becomes affected with disease
of the liver or kidneys. All these evils, although existing
in a temperate climate, prevail with double force in tropical
countries ; notably so in India, China, and the West Indies.
—*See* INTOXICATION.

DUTY.—*See also* GUARD.—In times of peace the *duties* of a soldier include his drills, parades, sentry or guard, picket, orderly, and so on. In times of war they are, of course, more arduous and at the same time more dangerous. There are then advanced and rear guards, it may be, duty in the trenches, and those directly against the enemy. In all cases it is necessary for a man's health that he have a good meal just before going on the particular duty; that his clothing be good and sufficient, and that he have means of keeping himself dry. If a man after a debauch goes upon severe duty, the chances are that he will be unfit for its performance, and that he will break down in his own health. Men should, as a matter of course, be permitted to perform the duties required of them with the least possible way, and without others being *tacked on.*

DYSENTERY is a frequent and fatal disease in damp hot climates, and in what are called "malarious" localities. In India, especially during and immediately after the rainy season, soldiers are very liable to its attacks. In temperate climates its virulence is comparatively rare, and its severity inconsiderable as compared to what they are abroad. So soon as a soldier is attacked with severe pain, increased on pressure, in the bowels, a feeling of weight and coldness there, frequent and ineffectual desire to go to the *rear*, he had better take hot drinks, as tea, apply hot fomentations, or a hot bottle, rolled in flannel to his stomach, and "report himself sick." Spirits are of no use in such cases. A little hot ginger or peppermint tea will give temporary relief, but the man must place himself without delay under regular medical treatment. Dysentery in the tropics is truly a fearful disease.

EARACHE.—This is a very common affection among soldiers, both at home and abroad. It is said to be caused in India by the use of punkahs and thermantodotes in barrack-rooms, and indeed, there are many persons, soldiers and others, who are unable to bear the use of either, even in the hottest weather. Earache is nothing more than inflammation of the inner parts of the ear, and requires to be treated like all other inflammations, that is, by hot fomentations and poultices. A man ought to apply one or other at once, or hold his face over the steam of hot water. The popular remedy of putting a piece of hot onion into the ear acts in the same way. The affection is a very painful one, and the person attacked with it had better report himself as soon as possible to the surgeon.

EDUCATION.—It is self-evident that the educated man has in many respects an advantage over the uneducated. This is so in all positions of life, but especially so in the army. In all nations, education of soldiers is looked upon as an important item in what constitutes military force, the soldiers who have sufficient learning to comprehend the object of particular movements and dispositions being obviously more likely to carry these out well, than those who merely obey orders mechanically, like so many machines. But education teaches, or ought to teach a man, not only his duty to his military superiors, but to his comrades and himself. It teaches him that there are other and greater pleasures to be attained than such as are of a mere bodily or material nature, and at the same time it affords the means of attaining them. What between schools and libraries provided for the soldier by Government, those who neglect to avail themselves of the benefits they are capable of affording have only themselves to blame. It has been well said, that "ignorance is the mother of error." Error thus arises in all that concerns a man, alike in relation to his bodily and moral state.

EMBARKING.—Full instructions in regard to the routine to be observed when troops are embarking for foreign service are contained in official *Regulations.* The duties which concern the health of the men include a careful inspection by medical officers, so that no person labouring under disease of an infectious nature shall proceed on board, that

sick and weakly men be left behind, and, in fact, that none
proceed except such as promise to be in every way efficient
for active or other service on reaching their destination.
This is necessary for the interests of the men themselves,
as well as for those of the public service. Soldiers when
about to embark should carefully avoid excess, or localities, where disease is rife, and where they may receive
the germs of maladies that may give rise to much suffering
and danger to life, not only during the sea passage, but after
arriving in the country to which they are proceeding. It is
necessary that men be amply provided with clothing and
other requirements before embarking, but their officers will
see that they are so.

EMETIC.—Sometimes a man feels that he requires an
emetic. He has taken some article of food that disagrees
with him, or perhaps swallowed by accident a morsel that
is "high," or otherwise offensive. He may have an illness
coming on, the first indication of which is a desire to get rid
of the contents of the stomach. The simplest plan for so
doing is to introduce one's own finger, or, better still, a
feather, into the mouth, and so tickle the throat. Many
persons have more or less the power to make efforts themselves to empty the stomach. By drinking a number of
glasses of warm water, one after another, vomiting will be
produced, and by continuing to do so the stomach may be
thoroughly and completely cleared out. This is the best
method to adopt, and the proceeding should be persisted in
till the end is gained.

ENDEMICS.—Particular localities and climates have their
peculiar *endemic* diseases, against each of which it is necessary to adopt precautions. In the United Kingdom, consumption and other diseases of the lungs, and rheumatism;
in India, cholera, liver, and dysentery ; in the West Indies,
yellow fever ; and so on. In all their habits and manner of
life, it would be well for soldiers if they considered what
are the particular diseases they have most to guard against

under the varying conditions of their service. In this way they would be the more likely to avoid them, and thus render the havoc caused in their ranks by *endemic* or climatorial disease fewer by far than they have hitherto been.

EPIDEMICS.—When these are raging, whether as cholera, yellow fever, or in other form, the best chance of escaping their onslaught is by being perfectly *clean* in person and sober in habits. Not that any human means known will always secure exemption from attack, but experience has amply shown that epidemics localise themselves and become intensified wherever filth prevails; persons weakened by debauch are thereby rendered doubly liable to attack, and when attacked have less chance of *pulling* through and making a complete recovery than those of more temperate and regular habits. The practice of drinking heavily "to keep off infection," so far from being beneficial, increases the liability to attack. The best plan is to make no change in the habits as regards food or drink, presuming them to be moderate, and to keep the mind and body, as far as possible, occupied. Men should never go upon duty while fasting.

EPILEPSY, OR FALLING SICKNESS.—A man is seized with an epileptic fit in the barrack-room. His comrades should take steps to prevent him from injuring himself during the convulsions which attend his fit. Open his clothes. Let him be placed in bed, upon his back, with chest and head a little raised. Sprinkle the face with cold water. When the fit is over, let the man sleep for a little; then be carried to hospital. The practice of forcibly restraining the limbs of a person in "a fit," ostensibly to prevent him from injuring himself, is improper, and often leads to the very evils it is meant to avert, dislocations of the joints and fractures of the bones being sometimes caused by it. The limbs should certainly be guarded, but so lightly and gently as to avoid the danger indicated. Sometimes the man affected threatens to bite his tongue or actually does so. It is best prevented by getting a roll of towel between his teeth.

EXERCISES.—These should be of duration and kind in proportion to the strength and capability of the individual. If necessarily violent they should be of short duration, and separated by time for complete repose. They are best undertaken in the morning and evening during summer ; in the middle of the day during winter. The more a soldier is kept actively employed the better fitted for war he remains, and the more healthy he is. After confinement in barracks or elsewhere, where the air is tainted, free exercise, by exciting the circulation and breathing, is best suited to enable him to *throw off* any evil effects that might afterwards arise. Walking, jumping, dancing, and gymnastics as conducted in regiments, are the exercises best suited to soldiers.

EYES, INFLAMMATION OF. SORE EYES, OR OPHTHALMIA. —In former days this disease often prevailed as an epidemic in regiments, Now, however, it is very rare indeed. Under the operation of unlimited service, there is every reason to believe that men used means to produce the disease in their own persons and to extend its prevalence in regiments, that they might obtain their discharge from the service. All this is, however, now changed. Inducements have ceased to act in leading men out of the army. Among the cáuses of sore eyes, two of the chief are overcrowding in barrack-rooms, and insufficient care in avoiding the promiscuous use of towels by the men. In India, especially, these causes operate. Another seems to be neglect as to bathing the eyes on returning to the barrack-room from parade, there being much reason to believe that the very fine dust with which the air is often loaded during the hot season, not only causes the disease itself, but conveys into the eyes various impurities which directly produce the affliction. The disease usually comes on suddenly. A soldier awakens in the morning and finds his eyelids swollen, his eyes hot and tender. There is nothing then to be done but to bathe them in hot water, and proceed to the hospital as soon as possible. The chief object in view should be to avoid the risk of attack by guarding against the causes enumerated. One kind of sore eyes—namely, *ulcerated cornea*—is often caused by neglect in the use of vegetables. A state of *scurvy* of the whole body thus arises, and the disease in question often arises as one of its consequences.

FAINTING.—Lay the fainting man in a current of fresh air, placing him at full length on his back. Do not raise his head. Undo his clothing over the neck and chest. Dash a little cold water over the face and chest. Place a scent-bottle, vinegar, or spirits under the nostrils for an instant. Repeat these measures at intervals of a few seconds, and if the *faint* is from ordinary causes the man will soon recover. If he does not recover, let him be carried at once to hospital. It is usually an easy matter to know when a man has fainted. He loses consciousness, falls, the breathing is scarcely visible; he lies as if dead, the face pale, the features "sharp," the nose pointed. A man may faint from being overheated, from being fatigued, from undertaking greater exertion than his strength is equal to, from having on too tight clothing or equipment, and from many other causes.

FALLING OUT.—There is often great injury to health produced by a soldier not falling out, or not being permitted to do so when necessity demands that he should. Men ought to be careful to make all their arrangements for parade so that they may in all likelihood not have to quit the ranks, as in many respects the practice is unseemly, besides being very annoying to the officers; nevertheless, when a sudden or urgent case of nature demands it, resistance is hurtful. No good soldier would of course make a practice of quitting his ranks while on parade, and no one would pretend to have to do so unless such were actually the case.

FATIGUE.—*See* REST.

FEET.—The feet of a soldier, especially of an infantry soldier, require great attention on his part to keep them in good condition, more particularly during continuous work. They should be kept clean. The toe nails should be cut, those of the great toes square, and clear of the *corners*, so as to prevent the risk of their growing into the flesh. On the march, the application of a little grease prevents *blisters* and *abrasions*; but at the end of each march the feet should be washed. In camp, and also in bivouac if possible, the feet should be left bare, or at any rate without boots during night. The application of brandy or of a little dry mustard in cold weather is recommended against the possible occurrence of chilblains, and then warm socks are indispensable. The French recommend a little spirits of camphor as an application when the feet are swollen or *frayed* by a long march. *See* BLISTERS. The feet must be kept dry and warm in order to prevent illness; especially colic, and " colds."

FIELD KIT.—The following is a list of the articles authorised to be taken by infantry soldiers when proceeding on the march or taking the field, in addition to what is worn on the person, viz. :—·

1 Pair of boots,
1 Pair of trousers,
1 Pair of mitts,
1 Pair of socks,
1 Shirt,
1 Towel,
1 Cap and badge,
1 Great coat,

1 Cloth brush,
1 Polishing brush,
1 Holdall complete,
1 Bible,
1 Tin of blacking,
Soap and sponge,
1 Small ledger-book,
1 Pot of grease.

It is usually so arranged as that one full set of brushes is carried among three men, each carrying one. The articles worn by the soldier include 1 chaco, 1 tunic, 1 shirt, 1 pair of trousers, 1 pair of braces, 1 pair of socks, 1 pair of leggings, 1 pair of boots, a clasp-knife and lanyard.

FIELD KITS FOR OFFICERS.—According to published lists they comprise the following, viz. :—Leather dressing-case,

D

with hair and clothes brushes, soap in metal box, nail brush, comb, and scissors, 18s.; 1 flannel shirt, 11s. 6d.; 1 pair of socks, 2s. 9d.; 1 pair of drawers, 6s. 8d.; 1 silk handkerchief, 4s. 9d.; 1 pair of shooting-boots, 38s.; 6 boot laces, at 6d. 3s.; 1 housewife, fitted, 6s.; cotton handkerchief, 8d.; sponge and bag, 6s. 6d.; great coat, grey waterproof, 136s. 6d.; uniform trousers, 42s.; cup, plate, knife, fork, spoon, pepper-box, salt, mustard, in leather case, 33s.; basin, india-rubber, or bucket, 7s.; plates, tin, at 4d. 8d.; book for writing, with ink, 7s. 6d.; vestas, box of, 6d.; mackintosh guard bed, 22s.; lamp, 4s. 6d.; regulation india-rubber waterproof cloak, 50s.; india-rubber ground sheet, 21s.; inflatable pillow, 8s. 6d.; inflatable bed, 21s.; canteen for three persons, 50s.; water bottle, 8s. 6d.; drinking cup-horn, 2s.; filter, 5s.; soap box, 2s.; cork mattress, covered with serge, 15s.; camp rug, 25s.; tent pole, hook, and straps, 3s.; night cap, 1s. 4d.; wooden bedstead with canvas bottom, 26s. 6d.; valise, 52s.; Colonel Wolseley's valise, as improved by Colonel Cochrane, is convenient for keeping the kit, and may be formed into a bed.

FILTERS.—*See* WATER.—It ought not to happen, with all our existing arrangements, that soldiers should often be without the means of obtaining good water. Circumstances may, nevertheless, occur when they are so. If that which they have to drink or cook with is muddy, stagnant, or containing fragments of decaying vegetable or animal matter, it should be filtered. This may be done in a simple way by pressing the handkerchief in it, or sinking it by means of a stone, and then drinking the water after it has passed through. A piece of flannel is better than ordinary linen cloth for the purpose. Another method adopted by travellers is if possible to make a small hole in the sand or mud at a little distance from the pool or ditch. The water will rise in it after passing through the intervening ground, and if permitted to rest for a little will be quite clear. Under general circumstances regular filters of one kind or another are provided by the proper authorities for camp and barracks.

FIRE.—*See also* COOKING. On service men may at times be thrown upon their own resources for lighting a fire, as for a good many other things. Their best plan is to dig a ditch or trench about twelve inches deep and broad and two feet or more long, or arrange logs of wood or bricks in the same position, the openings at each end being in the direction of the wind. *Firewood* should be cut in lengths of a foot long by two inches. Brushwood may be collected, or cow dung or bones used as fuel. With gunpowder, a flint and steel, some tinder and dry grass or twigs, a fire may for the most part be easily lighted, and now the *match-boxes* carried by almost every soldier afford ready means of doing so. Two hard stones struck against each other will produce sparks. Burning glasses, the lens of a telescope or binocular, will concentrate the sun's rays, and so produce fire in tinder or dry cotton.

FIRST DRESSING.—In the case of a soldier wounded in battle, the first dressing, such as may be applied by a comrade with the means each is supposed to carry on his person, and until the services of a surgeon can be obtained, should be directed with the view of securing the wound itself and its subject from injuries on the field or in transport to the rear. The wound should be covered to protect it from dust; if a limb is broken it should be gently placed in a proper and natural posture, and secured in that position. If there is bleeding, cloth or pads applied firmly to the wound may check the flow; but if not, and a man know the general course of the blood-vessels, he may be able to apply pressure with his fingers so as to stop it. If he does not know their course, a bandage or handkerchief should be tied tightly round the limb at a point nearer the body than the wound. The cloths applied to wounds upon the field should in all cases be first soaked in water, or in spirits and water if that be possible.

FISH.—The use of *stale* fish as food is often followed by signs more or less severe of poisoning, and very generally

D 2

by *nettle rash.* *Shell fish,* as oysters, muscles, &c., are at particular seasons and in some localities actually poisonous, and in tropical countries it is at all times unsafe to eat fish brought casually for sale, there being some that can never be eaten without risk. Under such circumstances it is never safe to *keep* fish overnight, even if soused with vinegar and spices. In India, *prawns,* and indeed every kind of "fish," are looked upon as likely to cause cholera in those who use them. Soldiers arriving in foreign countries should always be careful in respect to eating fish until they learn what are the kinds that are wholesome.

FLANNEL.—Some few persons suffer so much from irritation of the skin from wearing flannel, that they object to use it. Notwithstanding the inconvenience that is occasionally caused by it, however, it is indispensable for men engaged on service, undergoing fatigue, or having much exposure to the weather, as by absorbing perspiration, and being itself a non-conductor, it prevents the person from suffering from sudden chills, as he would do if he wore only cotton or linen. Statistics prove that on expeditions the men who wear flannel are less liable to sickness than those who neglect to do so ; mortality is also less among the former than the latter. During the winter season in cold or damp climates, the use of flannel underclothing is absolutely necessary for the preservation of health. By its use alone can men be protected against the diseases of the chest which are so prevalent during winter and early spring in Britain.

FOOD.—The soldier should carefully avoid committing errors in diet, or acts of debauch, as these not only destroy the healthy state of his digestion, but render him unable to perform his military duties. On the march or campaign he should not overload his stomach, neither should he use much salted or highly-seasoned meat, as these cause thirst, besides being hurtful in other ways. When on service or otherwise situated, so that the regular supply of food cannot always be depended upon, he should have in his haversack a small supply of some necessary articles, as biscuit, coffee, vinegar, and spirits. These would serve to render palatable such articles of food as might be obtained, and the three last diluted would serve as drinks or as fomentations. The French soldier considers that on service soups and stews form better modes of cooking meat than roasting. Hence they seldom adopt the latter, and perhaps they are right.

As a rule, the more agreeable food is to the sight and flavour, the more enjoyment there will be in eating it, the easier it will be digested, and the greater the good that will be derived from it. Food that is not relished, still more what is loathed, does no good, but, on the contrary, harm when eaten. The more severe the work to be performed, the larger the quantity of food required ; and soldiers on service, or about to go into battle, should have abundant and good food. Under all circumstances it is better to partake of food at short intervals than at long. In the latter there is risk of digestion becoming weakened, and in that state the stomach to be overloaded by too full a meal ; disease of the stomach may be caused in this way. Fresh meat is more nourishing than salted, but the latter occasionally as a variety is agreeable and wholesome. The amount and nature of food required are influenced to some extent by the *temperament* of the individual. The *sanguine* are believed to require relatively small quantities, but these must be nourishing of their kind ; for these, condiments, wine, and coffee are little needed. The *nervous* require a more varied diet, without stimulants. The *lymphatic* need a stimulant diet, as regards food and drinks. The *bilious* have always to exercise care as to what they eat and drink. Fat or *substantial* meat is for the most part injurious to them.

With regard to food in time of war, some points should be borne in mind by the soldiers themselves, as well as by the officers concerned. For the work then to be performed a pound of meat is considered to be required. Beef and mutton should as far as possible be given alternately, and in addition a portion of cheese is beneficial. Peas or beans are further excellent as articles of diet, as these supply the material (nitrogenous) which goes to form muscle. A certain quantity of fat is also requisite. It may be taken in the form of butter, or as bacon, the latter kind of food being especially suited for the duties a soldier has to perform. If the use of oil could be introduced into our army as it is in the armies of Continental Powers, it would form an excellent item of food taken with salads, and in other ways. Bread, when it can be obtained, is always preferable to biscuit. Potatoes and rice are good substitutes for bread. The use of salt is a necessity, and in cases where there is a deficiency of vegetables it has been recommended to use a small quantity of potash in addition to table salt, the potass being intended to supply the want of this salt, as it is one of the ingredients of vegetables. On service, and indeed at all times, the use of vinegar is very wholesome. It may be used with fresh salads or added to cold potatoes, carrots, &c., and is important as a preventive of scurvy.

Condiments of different kinds, such as sauces, pickles, mustard, pepper, &c., are not only grateful, but in moderation wholesome. Their use, too, makes all the difference between an insipid and a tasty meal.

The loss on meat by cutting up, bones, cooking, &c., is calculated at nearly one half of the original weight; thus one pound of meat in the raw state yields no more than half a pound actually to eat.

Salted pork or *beef*, or *smoked* meat are sometimes issued in place of fresh, on active service or on some foreign stations. When they are so, they must of course be of good quality, but it is, moreover, necessary that they be carefully and well cooked. The French recommend that when the salt meat is a little *high*, a little vinegar or a small piece of charcoal should be placed in the water in

which it is soaked prior to being cooked ; but inasmuch
as only the first quality of provisions are issued to the
British soldier, the precaution is doubtless unnecessary.
Bread should be well baked, well kneaded; the crust neither
too thick nor burned. *Biscuit* weight for weight is considered to be nearly double as nourishing as bread. Eaten
dry, it acts like a sponge, however, absorbing the fluids in
the stomach, and in the long run deranging digestion ;
hence, it should only be used continuously after being
soaked in coffee or in soup, after the manner of the French.
Rice should be white, little broken, and without much
flour. The grain of African and American is large ; that
of the Bengal small. *Preserved vegetables*, if issued, should
be " fresh " to the smell, and neither damp nor mouldy.
Potatoes should be firm to the feel, and not used after
they have begun to " shoot."

With regard to the actual quantities and kinds of articles
recommended to be used by the soldier as food on service,
the following are those laid down by Dr. De Chaumont,
namely:—Meat, with bone, 1 lb., or without bone, 12 ozs. ;
bread, 20 ozs. ; potatoes, 16 ozs. ; vegetables, as carrots, &c.,
4 ozs. ; peas, or beans, 3 ozs. ; cheese, 2 ozs. ; bacon, oil, or
butter, 2 ozs. ; sugar, 2 ozs. ; salt, ½ oz. ; vinegar, 2 ozs. ;
condiments as required ; tea, ½ oz. ; coffee, 2 ozs., or cocoa,
2 ozs.; making a total of 64 ozs. of solids. In addition, he
would allow 20 ozs. of beer, and 1 oz. of spirits, or 10 ozs.
of red French wine. This scale is excellent in every way,
and may with advantage be adopted by the soldier, or made
up in his articles of extra messing. The only point that
admits of doubt is in reference to the beer and the
spirits.

The following examples are given of the quantities of
food actually consumed by soldiers in England for the sake
of comparison, the total deductions from pay being also
made, alike for the quantities issued under the name of
Government Rations, and those issued as " Extra messing."
—*See also* RATIONS.

2ND BATTALION RIFLE BRIGADE.

Government Rations.

Bread, 1 lb. ; Meat, with bone, ¾ lb.

Stoppage on account of Government Rations, 4½d. per diem.

Extra Provisions.

Bread	½ lb.	Sugar	2 oz.
Flour every third or		Tea	1-6th oz.
soup day	½ oz.	Coffee	1-3rd oz.
Barley every third or		Mustard	1-12th oz.
soup day	½ oz.	Pepper	1-36th oz.
Potatoes	1¼ lb.	Salt	½ oz.
Other vegetables ...	1¾ oz.	Milk	1-8th pint
Butter...	3-14ths oz.		

Stoppage per diem for Extra Provisions, 3½d.

Total Consumed Daily.

Total solids   about   62 ounces.
   ,,   liquids   ...   ...   2 pints.
          Coffee, 1 pint.
          Tea, 1 pint.
          Soup, 1 pint every third day.
     (Soup days—Every third day.)

3RD DRAGOON GUARDS.

Government Rations.

Bread, 1 lb. ; Meat, with bone, ¾ lb.

Stoppage on account of Government Rations, 4½d. per diem.

Extra Provisions.

Bread	8 oz.	Sugar	2 oz.
Flour	0	Tea	1-5th oz.
Barley	0	Coffee	1-3rd oz.
Potatoes	1¼ lb.	Mustard	1-8th oz.
Other vegetables ...	2 oz.	Pepper	1-24th oz.
Butter	0	Salt	½ oz.
Cheese	0	Milk	2½ oz.

Stoppages per diem for Extra Provisions, 3½d.

Total Consumed Daily.

Total solids ...   ...   3 lb. 13 oz.
   ,,   liquids ...   ...   2¾ pints.
          Coffee, 1¼ pints.
          Tea, 1½ pints.

1st Brigade Royal Artillery.

Government Rations.

Bread, 1 lb. ; Meat, with bone, ¾ lb.

Stoppage per diem for Government Rations, 4½d.

Extra Provisions:

Bread ...	...	... 0	Sugar ...	...	...	3 oz.
Flour ...	...	... 4 oz.	Tea ...	...	...	¼ oz.
Barley ..	...	... 1 oz.	Coffee ...	...	...	1-3rd oz.
Potatoes	...	.. 1 lb.	Mustard	...	...	1-32nd oz.
Other vegetables	...	8 oz.	Pepper ...	...	:..	1-32nd oz.
Butter ...	...	... 0	Salt ...	...	...	1-16th oz.
Cheese ...	...	... 0	Milk ...	...	...	4 oz.

Beer, 1 pint daily.

Stoppage for Extra Provisions per diem, 4½d.

Total Consumed Daily.

Total solids ... ... 3 lb. 9 oz.
,, liquids ... ... 3 pints.
Tea, 1 pint.
Coffee, 1 pint.
Beer, 1 pint.

Roast meat, 3 days ; stewed, 3 days ; soup, 1 day per week.

With the introduction of the contemplated changes in regard to soldiers' pay, the daily stoppage of 4½d. for Government rations will cease.

FRACTURES.—*See* DISLOCATIONS.—This kind of injury may be *simple* or *compound*, that is, without or with a wound through the fleshy parts that cover the bone. *See also* WOUNDS *with* FRACTURES. Those that occur otherwise than in battle may be caused by blows, falls, by slips and accidents, at violent exercise, or in the gymnasium. The bones most liable to them are those of the limbs, the ribs, and *clavicle* or collar-bone. The signs of the accident, if in a limb, are swelling, unnatural appearance, impossibility on the part of the person to move the limb, great pain, and a grating sensation or *crepitus* when an attempt by a second party is made to move it. If the fracture be in the arm, it is possible that the patient may be able to walk to hospital. If in the lower, he must be carried. *See* STRETCHERS. To carry a man thus injured three *bearers* are requisite, and these should not only be prudent but calm and cautious. They should proceed to place him on a *stretcher* as described under that head, also that of CARRY-ING, being careful to avoid injury to the fractured limb, and so *carry* him to hospital. If a stretcher be from any cause not obtainable, a wheelbarrow having a thick bed of straw upon it may be used, or a cart similarly protected. Until the arrival of a surgeon all that can be done is to prevent the injured limb from being jerked and keep cold water applied to it.

FRUIT.—Like everything else, so in regard to fruit, a thing in itself good, when used in moderation, and at proper times, it becomes injurious when taken in excess or improperly. In temperate climates, and while no tendency to epidemic cholera or diarrhœa prevails, a soldier must in-deed take a very large quantity of fruit to do him harm. If he commit excess in this respect the chances are that he will suffer so severely from stomach-ache that he will not again run the same risks, and the less ripe the fruit is, the more severe will of course be the effects. In tropical climates, however, and especially in times of cholera, the use of fruit requires great caution, as in such cases, attacks of that disease, as well as of dysentery, are often directly pro-duced by it; and, moreover, there are in foreign countries many kinds of fruit very tempting to the eye which are yet very dangerous, some, indeed, actually poisonous in the use. The descriptions of fruit that are considered wholesome are usually allowed by commanding officers abroad to be taken round the barracks for sale, and to these soldiers should restrict themselves. In some cases, as when vege-tables are scarce or unprocurable, the use of the acid fruits is wholesome, in preventing the liability to *scurvy* that otherwise would arise. It is never safe for a soldier walking in a foreign country to pluck and eat any fruit he sees growing. Sometimes indiscretions of this kind are followed by very serious consequences so far as he himself is concerned.

FROST-BITE.—*See* COLD.—The parts " bitten " become at first red, then swollen and stiff, then white and insensible. They become cold, benumbed, and soon lose their vitality altogether. In such a state a man should not be brought into a hot room or near a fire, but should be left in an unwarmed room or the open air. He should be rubbed with snow on the spots affected, care being taken that violence is not used, otherwise the skin will get rubbed off. When circulation of the blood begins again in the frost-bitten parts the sensation of heat on the part of the patient becomes intense. Instead of continuing then to rub with snow alone, snow mixed with water may be used, the rubbing or friction being employed very gently indeed. If the frost-bite has been confined to the more exposed parts, as the face, nose, or ears, these should be very gently rubbed with a cold application at first, then after circulation has begun to return, with warm water and then with folds of dry cloth, being first smeared with oil. The further treatment must take place under the orders of the surgeon. To guard against frost-bite apply to the exposed parts of the body before going on duty during great cold, a little grease, or what is better, a little camphorated oil. Soldiers when serving in very cold climates or seasons should always provide themselves with either of these preparations. The ears are very liable to suffer in this way in severe winters. During the Franco-German war the soldiers of both armies were provided with woollen hoods which completely protected these parts. The hoods in question were called by the French, *passes montagnes.*

FUEL.—*On service,* the allowance of fuel is 3 lbs. of fire-wood or coals per man per day; with the latter, 1 lb. of kindling wood for every 36 lbs. of coal. This is only for cooking. The allowance of fuel on home service is obtained according to the following scale, per man, viz.: coal, 1 lb.; kindling wood, 6-7th lb., or turf, 1-112th kish. That for *cooking* is drawn separately. The allowance for this purpose varies according to the kind of cooking apparatus in use, and number for whom cooking is performed; as a rule, however, the strictest economy is needed to render the regular allowance sufficient.

FURLOUGH on sick certificate may be obtained by soldiers on home service on the recommendation of the surgeon-major of their regiment. When absent on such furlough, however, they must themselves bear the expense of medical attendance, except when they can obtain admittance into a military hospital. In all cases they should, if possible, refer to an army surgeon in the event of their desiring a renewal of their sick leave. It unfortunately so happens that from want of care and discretion on the part of men themselves, instead of those who obtain the indulgence for the benefit of their health really deriving any advantage from it, they are often seriously injured. Other men rush into recklessness of various kinds, and by no means seldom return to their regiments affected by *disease* of one kind or other, in addition to their original ailment.

GAITERS are happily not much worn in the British army. In the French, where they form an important item of the soldier's kit, they are far less useful than showy. They, and especially those of leather, contract the lower part of the leg, and when they become hard, as they do after long use and exposure to wet, they blister or *fray* the skin. If made to secure with buttons, these are apt to come off; they hurt the leg when marching, if made to *fit neatly*. If secured by laces, these get broken, and cannot be secured in a hurry or in the dark. The French surgeons saw all these disadvantages, and all are loud in their condemnation of the favourite gaiter, as being both useless and inconvenient. They advocate the substitution of the Prussian boot for the shoe and gaiter on active service.

GLANDERS.—The cases are infinitesimally few, still, soldiers of the English army do sometimes become attacked with this very fearful disease. The experiences in the late war on the Continent indicate that a few cases occurred among soldiers who had slept in or otherwise taken advantage of the shelter of strange stables, where diseased horses had no doubt been put up. Hence it is important to warn our own troops against making use of such places, should they be on the march or on service.

GRUMBLING.—A grumbling soldier is necessarily a discontented man. A habitually discontented man is sometimes led to commit excesses out of mere disappointment, rage, or other unworthy motive. Excesses, besides lowering moral character, expose a man to danger of accident and disease, and sooner or later lead to broken health. If, therefore, a soldier imagines he has cause of complaint in any way, let him seek an interview with his officer and respectfully tell him his grounds for thinking he has one. No good officer ever refuses to help a soldier, if it be in his power to do so. But if, as may so happen, the complaint is without sufficient grounds, or of a nature which cannot be immediately remedied, then the soldier should have the sense to put up with it for the time, knowing that if he does so, matters will in due time rectify themselves. Where, as in the army, strict rules are enforced for the good of the many, it cannot be but that in some instances they press hard upon an individual. If then he has patience, he may be sure that after a time *his luck will turn.*

GUARD.—Mounting guard is perhaps the duty that most constantly and continuously has to be performed by a soldier. Its frequent recurrence, by the mere fact of breaking and shortening his times of rest, has necessarily more or less of a wearing-out effect upon him. Hence the necessity on his part of not only doing nothing that is calculated to add to these effects, but of reducing as much as possible any inconvenience that may be unavoidable. It must be remembered that in all armies, guard duty, however inconvenient it may be to individuals, is looked upon as an important means of keeping troops in a state of military efficiency. It is the duty of commanding officers to reduce the number of guards, if possible, so that soldiers shall not have to mount, in a temperate climate, more than once in six days, and in hot climates, once in nine to twelve. Of course, there are many occasions when the *strength* of regiments does not admit of these rules being acted upon, but in India there exists an order, that whenever men are oftener on guard than once in three days a special report of the circumstance must be made to the authorities. During a soldier's tour of duty, he has sufficient opportunity between his turns of sentry to rest himself, and should accordingly avail himself of this spare time for the purpose. If the night be cold, he should avoid exposing the body or face to the heat of a fire before going on duty, as by so doing he renders himself more liable to catch cold. He should always have the means of changing socks or clothes that may become wet; and before mounting at night he should have a cup of good hot coffee. If he gets wet while on guard, it is obvious that he should change his clothes immediately he comes off, drying his wet ones at the fire in the guard-room.

GYMNASTICS.—These are regulated by special orders in regard to them. Yet the non-commissioned officers find the men themselves have it in their power to make some small but very important modifications. It is apparent that a young half-starved recruit, or one of lax and delicate fibre, will be unable to undergo exactly the same course as another whose condition is the opposite of all these. It is necessary that young lads should be *fed up* to enable them to undergo their regular course. Again, men are of different degrees of natural agility, and this fact should be borne in mind by instructors, as well as by men themselves while undergoing training. It must be evident also that the aptitude of a young man to perform particular feats must depend upon the occupation he followed previous to enlistment, and the muscles or limbs then most frequently employed in that occupation.

HABIT.—"Habit is second nature." The soldier, and especially while young, should guard against the risk of falling into habits which are neither good nor useful, which are expensive, and of a nature to cause inconvenience, if not absolute injury, to him in after years. Soldiers should remember that the age of early manhood is that in which the constitution most readily becomes accommodated to circumstances in which they may be placed, and also that in which habits and peculiarities are most readily contracted. They should therefore accustom themselves to cleanliness, activity, sobriety in all things, to regular method, and to the virtue of living upon their means. Those who begin their career by recklessness find it very difficult after a little to *pull up*.

HÆMORRHAGE.—*See* WOUNDS WITH MUCH BLEEDING.—In order to check hæmorrhage from a large vessel, pressure in some shape or other must be used, as by means of wetted pads, or the fingers, or the application of a handkerchief above the part, a piece of wood being placed under it and the cloth twisted tightly, so as to check the flow of blood towards the injury. In all cases where a wound is bleeding freely the utmost haste should be used in sending for a medical officer, as the life of the patient must always be looked upon as in the utmost danger. There is a particular habit of body in which slight wounds, as scratches, having a tooth out, and so on, are followed by inordinate and even dangerous bleeding. Cases of this peculiarity are very rare, but when they do happen they require the attention of the surgeon.

HANGING.—In some rare instances an unfortunate man attempts suicide by hanging. This, when it happens, takes place usually in a prison cell. The body is to be immediately cut down, the cord undone and removed from the neck. He should then be carried to a place where there is plenty of fresh air, laid upon his back with the chest slightly raised, and treated precisely as if for recovery from DROWNING. Cold water should be applied to the head.

HEAD.—Should be kept *clean* by daily brushing and combing the hair, and by frequent and thorough washing with soap and water. Regulations restrict the length of the hair, but, irrespective of them, the shorter the hair is kept the more easily kept clean it is. Every man should use a small-tooth comb. No man ought to use his neighbour's hair-brush, as very nasty and obstinate diseases of the skin are sometimes spread in this way. Of course, the brush used should be itself clean.

HEALTH, the greatest blessing, is that which all men are most liable to lose, whether by causes over which they have no control, or by such as might be avoided. Soldiers are, from the nature of their profession, subject to some causes of loss of health which do not affect the civil population. In addition to these, they destroy it by excesses of different kinds—drink, libertinage, late hours, and indulgences in other ways; they injure health by errors in regard to food, clothing, and from errors in other ways, committed through ignorance or thoughtlessness. Health is influenced by the various conditions under which we live; by air, temperature, and climate; by accommodation, food, clothing, nature of work; by rest and exercise; by exposure or otherwise to epidemic influences; and, to some extent, at least, by the class of places we visit and of persons we associate with. In fact, it may be said that health, cleanliness, and morality go hand in hand.

HEALTH. PRESERVATION OF.—During the Franco-German war, distinct codes of instructions for the preservation of health were issued by the respective Governments for the use of their soldiers. Nor can we do better than transcribe the following, found on the person of a Prussian soldier killed in battle :—

"We know by experience in all wars that our incomparable soldiers suffer much more by disease than by the risks of wounds and death in battle, yet a great many of the diseases may be avoided by care, attention, and foresight. Nothing can be more dangerous than to believe too much in one's own strength. If many of our soldiers fall sick during war it is by over-eating and want of cleanliness. By these two evils the country often loses heroes who have escaped the bullets and sabres of the enemy. For these reasons the soldiers, but still more the officers, should actively see to the execution of the following rules :—

" 1. The soldier should drink for thirst fresh and pure water. On the march and in hot weather it is impossible altogether to abstain from drinking, but it is necessary to be careful, and especially about the water used. Drink little by little, without swallowing the first few mouthfuls ; these should be thrown out and the temples at the same time be wetted.

" If there is no well or cistern water, but only that of rivers, tank, or ditch, it should, if possible, be filtered through charcoal, or it should be boiled, then allowed to cool, and afterwards mixed with brandy, tea, or coffee.

" 3. To drink pure brandy, rum, or other spirits in order to quench thirst is bad, because these reproduce thirst, and instead of strengthening, weaken the person.

" 4. The soldiers should never drink beer that is ' turned,' cider, nor wine of the country to which they have not previously been accustomed, even if they are offered, as they induce pain and derangement in the stomach and bowels.

" 5. Tea and coffee are, it is true, very light drinks for fatigue : they are better than water however ; they can be drank cold, are prepared in the early morning and carried in the water bottle with which each soldier is furnished. A slice of lemon or a little vinegar may be added, if the weather is hot.

" 6. Often the soldiers are hungry and thirsty. When they find fruit and grapes they think these will satisfy them, but they will not ; they are cold, they only increase the hunger and the thirst, and themselves cause inconvenience.

" 7. If mouldy bread be offered the mouldy part should

E

be cut off and the remaining part heated. Baking or heating will destroy the mouldy taste.

" 8. Fresh cooked food, especially potatoes, is best for the nourishment of the soldier.

" 9. Fresh meat should only be roasted for a short time; it should not be eaten too much cooked; if boiled, it should be at once put into hot water so as to preserve the juices. As to salted meat, it should be steeped for some time in warm water before being cooked.

" 10. One great matter for the preservation of health is cleanliness of the body as well as of the linen and clothes. The men should bathe when warm, and especially the feet and eyes; these should also be bathed in the morning and again at night before going to bed.

" 11. The feet should be maintained carefully in a state of cleanliness. Care should be taken to grease the boots if they become hard; the inside should be rubbed with soap and suet. If the feet are sore, change the socks often. Bands of linen are better than socks, because they can more frequently be washed. To heal blisters, drop upon them a little brandy or warm suet.

" 12. Many diseases arise from cold, because the young soldiers do not cover themselves sufficiently. Cotton or flannel shirts are, in such a case, preferable to those of linen. Men whose chests are weak should wear flannel shirts or woollen waistcoats. For affections in the abdomen a woollen belt is excellent.

" 13. When the soldiers enter their quarters they should immediately close the windows and avoid draughts of air.*

" 14. In marching during hot weather they should cover the head and neck with a light linen cloth, as for example, a pocket handkerchief, and should put a fine net over the mouth, so as to guard against thirst.

" 15. On being attacked with the slightest illness it is

---

* Surely this is a little too absolute. Fresh air, so long as there is no direct draught can do no harm.

recommended that the soldier show himself to the medical
officer; many, from pride or bashfulness, avoid doing so
until too late, and after the attacks, at first light, as ca-
tarrhs, diarrhœa, and so on have degenerated into sources
of danger."

HEAT APOPLEXY.—*See also* APOPLEXY.—In India, during
the hot winds, a man is found, perhaps in the guard-room
or cells where he has been confined, in his bed in barracks
or hospital, lying upon his back in a state of insensibility,
with stertorous breathing or heavy snoring, froth issuing
from the mouth or nostrils, the face generally greatly
flushed, the whole surface of the body red, intensely hot,
and especially so over the pit of the stomach. If the
hand be placed on that part, a thrill of heat of a very
peculiar and distinctive character will be felt. Sometimes
the patient moans, or talks at intervals incoherently;
sometimes he moves his arms about, or strikes them
against his own person. Generally, however, he lies perfectly still upon his back. In such a case, if dressed, the
clothing should be stripped off. At any rate, the patient
should be at once completely soused with water thrown
from a height; one stream directed upon his head, care
being taken that his mouth and nostrils are kept clear of
the stream for respiration; another should be directed over
the pit of the stomach. It is well to be careful that the
head is properly supported, as by its being in an awkward
position, so that the chin presses against the chest, breathing may be rendered impossible, and the patient thus suffo-
cated. As soon as a stretcher has been got, carry the man
to hospital, his whole body covered with *wet clothes.* In
India—as, for example, during the Mutiny campaign—it
was found that men and officers had every now and then
to have water poured over them, and march along until they
became dry again. In this way, heat apoplexy was averted.
It is also necessary, under such circumstances, to avoid
over-indulgence in beer or spirits. It is usually the dissipated who become the subjects of this affection.

E 2

HEART, DISEASE OF.—This class of diseases have, unfortunately, become very prevalent in the army of late years, and much attention has been bestowed by surgeons on their investigation. They seem to be induced by a combination of causes, rather than by any one ; and whether they be what are called *organic*, or merely functional, are alike grounds for discharging their subject from the service, although in the latter case their presence does not unfit him for work in civil life, nor necessarily shorten his life. The best means of guarding against their occurrence are the following :—The young recruit to be not over-drilled; not too long kept in a constrained attitude; to be encouraged to spend his surplus money more in the purchase of eatables than drinkables ; to be put on his guard against *excesses*. The practice of soldiers—old as well as young—remaining in public-houses so late that they have to run, probably up-hill, so as to be in time for the *last post*, is, it is to be feared, a fertile source of these affections. They are stuffed and stuffy from eating, drinking, and smoking, and thus soon get *winded* when they have run short distances. In some constitutions, tobacco-smoking seems undoubtedly to cause a liability to these affections, and it certainly aggravates them when they occur.

HORSE-FLESH.—The use of horse-flesh as food is repulsive to the ideas of British soldiers. The French, however, use it freely, and after a battle are thus enabled to make very hearty meals, when otherwise they would be badly off. There is cause to believe that it is unsuited for continued use, but that is no good reason why it should not be partaken of if such a necessity should arise. The French convert it into soup when bivouacking on the field, and thicken the bouillon with biscuit.

HUTS.—Various kinds of huts are used for accommodating troops. That most convenient for war service is the *Glo'ster* hut, 28 feet long, 16 feet wide, 6 feet high at

the eaves, 16 feet at the ridge, and capable of holding
24 men. Another kind of hut is erected, each capable of
holding 28 men. These are 32 feet long, 16 feet broad, and
6 feet high from slope to wall plate. Two of these may
be put up end to end, separated by a partition wall containing the fireplaces. Mud huts can be thrown up. Thus
the Sardinian soldiers in the Crimea took advantage of
inequalities of ground to make huts, the roof sloping down
from the scarped face of a ridge; the gables made by loose
stones. One of this kind, 14 feet 3 inches long, and 7 feet
1 inch wide, accommodated 6 men. In India, the "temporary" barracks erected at many places, as, for example,
when the Punjaub was first occupied, and during the
Mutiny were nothing more than huts consisting of wood
and mud. These have given way to more imposing buildings now, but there was a time when they existed at almost
every station throughout the country. During the late
war in France huts of various kinds were quickly run up
for the troops employed in besieging cities, as also for those
defending them. In this country the huts in the "camps"
are certainly cold in winter, but it may be consolatory to
the soldier to know that they are healthy, even in the case
of men arriving at these places from hot countries. In
fact, the *malaria* they bring in their systems seems to be
thus dispelled.

HYGIENE.—The science so called, that of preserving
health, derives its name from *Hygieia*, the daughter, according to old Greek mythology, of Esculapius. Esculapius
was also called *the life-giver*, his daughter Hygieia, *the
health-giver;* and we learn that in those ancient times quite
as great a degree of importance was assigned to the preservation of health as to the art by which it was recovered
when lost. As applied to soldiers, hygiene derives a degree
of importance far greater than it does in civil life, and thus
its practice becomes a speciality. In civil life it is true
that the interests of the individual and of the public have

alike to be considered. In addition to these, however, other considerations of great moment have to be taken into account in applying the science in the army. Soldiers have always been and now more than ever are the real *sinews* of war; the commander who is able to bring the largest number of efficient men to bear upon a given point at a particular time is he with whom success declares. itself. In order, therefore, that soldiers by whom virtually battles are fought shall be physically prepared for the fight, they must be as far as practicable preserved from the known causes of disease, the strength of the healthy main-- tained, the duration of unavoidable sickness and of wounds shortened to the utmost. The medical officers of the army have to study the varying conditions demanded by military service, and devise means best calculated to pre- serve health under all of them; yet it must be obvious that to a very considerable extent much of the success of those measures depends upon the soldier himself, towards whom they are specially directed. Unless individual men carry out, each for himself, the rules that alone can ensure- health and efficiency, such rules, however good and suit-- able in themselves, will be ineffectual to secure the great end they have in view.

ILLNESS.—It does not comport with the position of a. soldier to have a constant dread of illness, and to be always under apprehension of attack. On the other hand, it is equally injurious to *brave* the first seizure of disease, there- being many which, although easily combated in their early shapes, yet if left to themselves speedily become uncontrol- lable. Therefore, a soldier ought to lose no time, when fairly ill, in applying for medical aid. The idea of *shaking off* grave disease is simply foolish. As well might a man hope to *shake off* mortality. Often a little rest and quiet in. hospital for a few days, will of itself be sufficient to ward off what would, if unattended to, become an attack of illness, provided this be attended to sufficiently early.

INDIA.—A special paragraph is given to *India*, the more distinctly to impress upon men and officers the necessity, for some time at least after arriving in that country, to beware of the risks they run, not only from endemic diseases of the country, but from the effects of any recklessness or indiscretions of which they may be guilty. Experience, often gained under painful circumstances, has led all classes who have lived some years there to adopt certain habits and style of dress, to keep certain hours different from those observed in England, and to adapt themselves in a great variety of ways to the conditions of the climate. It is a common thing for the newly-arrived regiments, men and officers, to pretend to ignore all those habits, to keep up those of home. The consequences soon manifest themselves. Sickness and death begin to rage, an epidemic of cholera takes place, the survivors are sent home to England " sick ;" and by-and-bye routine is adopted such as circumstances have made compulsory on every regiment that has ever served in India, and which would have been the means of saving many a life in each of them if that routine had been adopted earlier. Persons who have little or no practical experience of India, may say what they choose as to the country being *healthy* if it were not for the *indiscretions* on the part of those who suffer and die there. The facts remain that the climate is as unhealthy as it is unnatural to a native of Britain, and that care is ever necessary, so that the subtle influences of disease may be in some degree, if not altogether counteracted.

INFECTION.—There exists a very general, and, it must be added, well-grounded dread of *infection;* hence the unlucky man who becomes the subject of small-pox, scarlet fever, or other disease that is capable of being propagated in this way, must be prepared to be placed in quarantine, and have communication between him and his friends completely cut off. This is most necessary in regiments, where the greatest good of the greatest number has to be considered rather than individual interests. Nevertheless, it may be well to observe that there really exists less danger of a person visiting a patient affected with such diseases becoming himself attacked with them than many people suppose. The actual sphere within which infection acts is comparatively limited, always assuming that the visitor does not breathe the breath of the patient, or the emanations given out by his body. It is essential, however, for his own safety, that the visitor be in good health, perfectly clean, and perfectly sober. An individual may, without himself being the subject of infectious disease, convey and propagate the infection by means of his clothes. Some persons, also, are more liable than others to " catch" infection.

INFIRMIERS ; *i.e.*, ORDERLIES over Sick or Wounded.— The functions of an attendant upon the sick have an importance second only to those of the medical officer. In several respects the question of the life or death of a patient is resolved by the fitness or unfitness of the *infirmier ;* it is, therefore, a matter of the utmost importance that men selected in that capacity should be qualified for it, and fully conscious of the important part it is their duty to fulfil. It is above all things necessary that they should guard against that *hardness* which is said to become engendered by familiarity with suffering. They should be respectable men, of tolerable education, affable and kind to the patient, watchful at all times, but especially at night, and careful to carry out the orders of the surgeon, in spirit at least, if not to the letter. In all armies the desire is to obtain the most respectable men as *infirmiers.* In that of Germany special inducements are held out for soldiers in this position to adopt nursing as a profession, those who obtain certificates of qualifications from the medical officers being pretty sure of employment in civil hospitals, asylums, &c., after having completed their military service.

INTOXICATION—*See* DRUNKENNESS.—In the greater number of cases all that is necessary is to place the person in such a position that as he lies there shall be no risk of suffocation. Thus, let his head and shoulders be gently raised; then sponge or sprinkle his face with cold water, and allow sleep to recover him. In very bad cases, where the patient threatens to die, proceed as in that of a drowning man. *See* DROWNING. Move him gently from side to side. Endeavour to produce vomiting. Apply strong scents to the nostrils. Rub the limbs. Bathe the face with cold water, or water containing spirits or vinegar. If a man insensible from intoxication is placed in a solitary cell, he should be visited at short intervals by the sergeant of the guard, otherwise he may turn himself into such a position as to be unable to breathe, and thus die by suffocation.

LIGHT.—Without free exposure to the light of the *sun,* health and strength alike suffer. Children brought up in close streets and alleys are for the most part sickly, often morally as well as physically debased. Light is as necessary for the full health of a man as it is for that of a plant, and without it both alike become *bleached.* Barracks in temperate climates are built so as to receive the greatest amount of light; so are hospitals, and any soldier who has been ill is aware of the pleasure felt when he for the first time is able to leave his bed and fairly enjoy the sunlight. Cheerfulness is encouraged by light, and depression by the absence of it. *Consumption* is one of the diseases that are induced by the absence of light.

LIGHTNING.—A man is struck by lightning. Let him be laid in an open place, where he can have free circulation of air, undressed, and his whole body sponged with cold water. Rub his arms and legs; tickle his nostrils. The limbs that are insensible should be wrapped in linen or cotton cloth moistened with spirits and water; the parts that are burnt, smeared with oil. If the man be delirious, or there are convulsive movements of the limbs, the head is to be freely bathed with cold water. Artificial respiration may be tried, as in the case of drowning, and as soon as the patient is able to swallow he should have a little spirits given to him.

LIVER.—Disease of the liver is almost exclusively confined to soldiers serving in the East and West Indies. It is most common in the former. Undoubtedly, over-eating, over-drinking, and needless exposure, whether by night or day, are among the more frequent causes; yet it is well that the steady soldier should know that even he is by no means exempt, the continued heat of the climate being often capable of producing the affection. Sometimes the attack is sudden, the person being seized with excruciating pain under the right ribs; sometimes it comes on more gradually, with a general feeling of being out of sorts, want of appetite, feeling of heaviness in the side and constipation. Once the disease has really become confirmed, it is seldom got rid of in India. The only advice, therefore, that can be given, is—Take it in time; consult your medical officer, and trustfully submit to the treatment prescribed by him.

LOADS.—A soldier may often be so situated as to require to extemporize carriage for stores of different kinds, and therefore he should know what weights may be carried by the different means employed. A donkey will carry about 60 lbs., a small mule 100 lbs., a horse 200 lbs., an ox 200 lbs., a camel 400 lbs. An animal, except a camel, will draw upon wheels about twice and a half the weight he will carry. A light cart, exclusive of the driver, should not carry more than 800 lbs.; a light waggon, with one or two horses, 1,500 lbs.; and a waggon of the strongest construction not more than 3,000 lbs. As to the quantity of food forming loads, a strong waggon will carry 1,000 full day's rations.

LOST.—If you lose your road in the dark, the best plan is to remain where you are till daylight, making what protection you can against attacks by wild beasts. If you lose your way in the daytime, proceed in such a way as to leave marks of your course ; mark twigs of trees, or drag a stick to make a track. If you see smoke, even at a great distance, make for it. If in a desert or large plain you lose your way, and also lose count of direction, your plan is not to wander, but remain in one place, in the hope of sooner or later being relieved. In India, the frequent occurrence of sunken wells, without any fence round them, renders it extremely dangerous for soldiers to wander about at night, and many lives used to be lost by men falling down them.

LUNGS.—These organs are extremely liable to become diseased in the United Kingdom. Disability from this cause is very common among soldiers, young and old. Much may be done by men themselves to guard against disease, or to delay the development of those germs that are inherited by them from their parents. The more violent the exertion undertaken, or the more rapid a pace at which a soldier walks, the more rapid his respiration will be, and the more work is thrown upon the lungs. Exposure to wet and chills on the one hand, and neglect of proper ventilation in the barrack-rooms, increase the risks of these diseases. So does want of care in regard to clothing. A man becomes hot : he throws open his dress ; it may be stands in a draught, or perhaps lies down on the damp grass. The natural result is an attack of *cold*, or inflammation on the lungs, from which recovery may perhaps be difficult. When a soldier does become thus affected, the sooner he consults his medical officer the better for himself.

MALARIA.—The presence of the influence so named is doubtless the actual cause of ague, and other fevers of various kinds. It is always most powerful in its action at night, and indeed is for the time being rendered powerless by dry heat of 868 F. and upwards. If troops have to halt during the night in a malarious locality, they should know that by lighting fires between them and the place whence it arises, or around them, they afford themselves the best protection in their power against it. If passing through such places a pocket handkerchief applied to the nostrils so as to admit of breathing taking place through it, is also in some measure a safeguard, as the *malaria* clings to vegetable fibres. Whatever be the actual nature of malaria or *marsh miasma*, practical experience proves that it is most powerful in its effects in low damp localities, the soil of which consists of rich mould or alluvium; that in such localities intermittent fevers or ague prevail in temperate climates, and in addition remittent or jungle fever, diarrhœa, dysentery, and cholera, in hot and tropical climates. All marshes, however, do not produce malaria; thus the *peat bogs* of Ireland and Scotland are free from it. In some countries, more especially in those that are tropical, the act of turning up the soil liberates malaria, hence the obvious necessity of avoiding to do so when pitching camps or individual tents. If soldiers are obliged to sleep or remain in a malarious locality, in addition to using the precautions already indicated, they should keep the doors of their huts or tents closed on the side facing the source of it, use no water except what is filtered, take a little *spirits*, wine, or malt liquor, and be careful to have some hot coffee before quitting camp in the early morning. QUININE WINE is also useful as a preventive.

MALINGERING—FEIGNING ILLNESS—in olden days used to be very common among soldiers. It is now comparatively rare. The ease with which inefficient men may be replaced makes it of little account to retain either the unhealthy or the unwilling. It is a mistake on the part of the malingerer, however, to suppose that his fictitious illness passes undetected by the surgeon and his comrades. Often the former, even when he does not appear to be so, is quite aware of the imposition, but as the impostor is for the most part a man of bad character, everybody is glad to get rid of him. There can be no meaner conduct than for a person to pretend being ill when he is not, thus practising deception and throwing extra duty upon the more honest of his comrades.

MARCH.—Order and precision on the line of march have also their influence upon health. It is the duty of officers to see that the time selected for the march shall, if the requirements of the service permit, be such as to avoid the great heat of the sun in summer or tropics, and the greatest cold in winter. The troops should never begin a march until after they have broken their fast in some manner, say by a cup of coffee and a biscuit. Officers will see that the rate of pace is moderate, and that *spurts* are avoided, that the proper distances between files, ranks, and larger bodies is maintained; that the halts are neither too long, nor in positions where the men, heated with exertion, shall be exposed to draughts of cold wind. No man should stray away from the column. Whenever a halt of sufficient length takes place, it is well to take off the boots and socks, dust them, and wash the feet in cold or tepid water, bathing the eyes and face at the same time. Our soldiers, while pursuing the mutineers in India in 1857 and 1858, had often to march throughout the heat of the day, and during the hot winds. They every now and then soaked their heads and whole bodies in water, carried for the purpose in skins on the backs of elephants, camels, &c., and thus were enabled to continue their journey, APOPLEXY being at the same time averted. To drink much while on the march is injurious, even if it be only of water. Spirits or beer to excess simply render a man unfit to march. Doubtless the reputed cases of APOPLEXY among troops in the United Kingdom are in reality from the effects of over-drinking. The collar and breast of the tunic should always be open during long or quick marches. In Europe the regular roads are considered those best suited for marching upon. In India the *cutcha* or unmetalled roads, although very dusty, are preferred by the troops. The men themselves soon find how necessary it is in India so to time the hour of starting that they shall reach their new camp ground before the sun becomes hot. They also soon learn how necessary and enjoyable is the half hour's halt midway, and the coffee and biscuit then served out to them, generally just as day is breaking. If a *malarious* track of country has to be traversed, the officers in command, on the recommendation of the medical officer, will see that marches take place while the sun is up, provided circumstances admit of this. In some books allusion is made to the supposed advantage of men while marching having their toes either turned a little in, or at any rate the feet not being turned outward. The best plan seems to be to retain the position in this respect to which individual men have been accustomed. Officers should see that on the line of march troops occupy their proper side of the road. Thus, horses and conveyances meeting or passing them do not cause inconvenience. They should also avoid having the men under arms for a needlessly long time before the march begins. The pace should at first be moderate, afterwards accelerated, and again slow before reaching the camping ground. It is considered advisable to have a short halt every hour, and a long halt midway; and for obvious reasons the midway halt should be longer than any of the others. On these occasions the men should not be harassed by orders of a trifling nature, the object being to give them as much rest as circumstances permit. Men on a long march soon come to suit their hours of sleep to the time they have to begin their march. Regular hours are very necessary, and care should be taken by their commanders and others not to disturb unnecessarily the men who are asleep. It is well known that the men become more fatigued the nearer they are to the rear of a column on the march. Hence the propriety of changing the order of march in that respect from day to day.

MARRIAGE.—Considering the changes in the military system now contemplated, marriages *with leave* will soon virtually cease among soldiers under the colours. As, however, men will have passed through their period of active service by the time they attain the age of 26, this is not only no real hardship, but a direct advantage to them, whether they think so or not. In former days when soldiers remained 21 years and more in the ranks, those who were married were amongst the most steady and respectable in the regiment, as well as those most exempt from sickness, and consequently most efficient as soldiers ; yet as their means were very seldom sufficient to keep their wives and children, these had to undergo trials and privations of a very sad kind. often bringing with them great anxiety and unhappiness to the husband. During marches and on board TRANSPORT SHIPS the families of soldiers used to suffer great discomforts; during active service wives and children had to be left with only the small provision made for them by Government, and depending upon such charity as well-disposed people chose to bestow for their assistance. Taking all these things, therefore, into account, I would say to a soldier about to marry. Decidedly " don't " while in the ranks as a private. Marriages contracted " without leave " cannot be too strongly condemned. A soldier in this state must either act like a villain and cast off his wife, or reduce her and himself to abject poverty. They must take lodgings in the lowest and very worst localities in garrison towns, in the midst of crime, where vice abounds, and to one or other or both of which they will very probably sooner or later fall victims. Women who marry under such circumstances are not as a rule desirable in any way as wives, but rather the very opposite. It may be added that little do young women who are on the look out for soldiers on Sunday afternoons know how miserable is the position of a soldier's wife under many conditions, notwithstanding that certainly much is done with a view to enhance their comfort.

MORALITY.—The soldier who leads a life of morality and self-restraint is he who enjoys the soundest health, is best fitted for duty, is most likely to gain promotion, and to obtain a pension sufficient to keep him in ease during old age.   There are still higher objects than these to be looked for from a life of morality.   The reckless and immoral make the worst soldiers ; those who enter battle with a full knowledge of their condition are always the most trusted, and the most likely to be victorious.—*See* BATTLE.

NAILS.—Soldiers require to keep the nails short.   In cutting those of the great toe, they should leave them *square* at the sides.   They will thus grow clear of the skin there, and avoid giving rise to the painful affection caused partly by the practice of cutting them too short, and wearing boots that are too tight over the part.   *In-growing nail* is best treated by softening the nail by means of a poultice, then scraping it with a penknife, or piece of glass, until so thin at the edge that it becomes flexible ; a small piece of cotton, sponge, or other soft material, should then be gently pressed under the embedded corner, and being renewed daily, a cure may be effected without the soldier having to go to hospital.

NIGHT.—Not only are men more liable to become attacked by illness at night from the fact of their own vital forces being less strong than during day, but the condition of the air is such that the influences of disease are more extensively prevalent than during daytime.   Besides this, except when men are on duty, those who are out at night are, for the most part, after no good.

NOSE, BLEEDING FROM.—This is by no means uncommon among young soldiers.   If slight, all that is needed is to bathe the face and nose with cold water, and in fact, a little bleeding of this kind not only is at times of no harm, but often actually an advantage, especially when there is " fulness of the head " present.   If it continues long, or is to a great extent, the dress should be *undone*, the person laid upon the ground; his head and face bathed, or *rinsed* with cold water, or spirits and water if they can be got.   As it usually takes place, however, it is without any great danger to the person affected by it.

OFFICERS.—It would be well for individuals and for the interests of the service if the intercourse between soldiers and officers in the army were more intimate than it is. On active service common risks and common hardships bind them together to a certain extent, but, as a rule, the *genius* of both, and the circumstances of barrack life are adverse to the continuance of feelings so engendered. Perhaps these pages may be read by officers. If so, I would point out to them that soldiers are great discriminators of character, that they are sensitive of neglect or injury real or supposed, and equally so of consideration towards them. Considering also the relative position of officers and soldiers, the power left in the hands of the former, the powerlessness of the latter, it is nothing less than dastardly to treat them in a way that would be instantly resented by a man in civil life, however low his social position. The demeanour of the soldier towards his officer must at all times, and under all circumstances, be respectful, and that of the latter to him should always be considerate; for who has the soldier to whom he may look for help and guidance, if it be not his officer? Strictness on duty is quite compatible with urbanity.

ORDERLIES.—*See* INFIRMIERS.

PARADES.—*See also* DRILLS.—It is only on parade that soldiers can learn their duty. Their officers know that short and frequent parades fatigue and harass them less than such as are long and tedious. The one interests, the other wearies. The individual soldier, before going on parade, should be prepared in every way, so that he may, if possible, avoid *falling out*. He should, if health be considered, have a meal of some kind, as a cup of tea and a slice of bread, before early morning parade. If heated on parade, he should be careful on returning to barracks to

F

avoid exposing himself to a draught, or standing in the passages partially undressed.

PASSIONS.—A soldier who is unable to control or command his passions, if there be such a person, can hardly be considered to have reached the condition of a man. His mental development is below that of many of the so-called lower animals, inasmuch as the latter can, to a certain degree, exert control over theirs. Let a man ask himself what he gains by absence of this control. Sudden rage leads to crimes of violence; these to punishment and degradation. Indulgence in vice, to disease, permanent ill-health, inability to work, and hence to all the miseries of poverty. Are a few so-called pleasures worth such risks? Let each man ask himself the question. He may depend upon it that a steady quiet life, if less exciting than one of scrapes and self-indulgence, ensures far greater personal comfort, and the chances of health, as well as advance in his profession. True, the *fast* soldier sometimes reforms. The sooner he does so the better for his own health and well-being. The opinion cannot be permitted to remain unchallenged that a man cannot command himself if he but resolutely make the attempt. Of course he can.

PEMMICAN.—This preparation of meat is used by sailors in arctic voyages, by sportsmen in various countries, and may, under special circumstances of service, have to be so by soldiers. It consists of a mixture of 5-9ths of dried and pounded meat to 4-9ths of melted or pounded fat put into a bag or box while somewhat warm. Sometimes wild berries are added to it. This becomes so hard as to require to be cut with an axe. It is at first unsightly in appearance; but men soon become accustomed to that, and then it furnishes an excellent article of food. It is said to be a wholesome food, and under the conditions in which it is for the most part used, is certainly a great boon.

PERSPIRATION.—Not only does perspiration, if cleanliness

be not observed, become extremely offensive to the companions of a soldier, but it soon becomes injurious to his own health and to that of others in the same barrack-room with him. The matters thrown off from the body soon decompose, and unless removed from the body become literally an enveloping layer of rotting animal substances, at the same time that they fill up the pores in the skin by which the natural secretions of it would otherwise escape. As soon, therefore, as possible, a man who returns to barracks perspiring freely should have a good bath of soap and water. He should lay out his clothes to dry in the sun or near a fire. It is the neglect of such precautions that renders intercourse with the multitude of "the great unwashed" so extremely unpleasant to persons of delicate senses.

POISONING.—It is not often that a soldier swallows a poison. When he does however, his comrades should use such means as may be available to prevent, as far as possible, its taking effect. The first thing to be done is to induce vomiting if possible, as by giving warm water—whether salt or fresh—to drink, or tickling the throat with a feather. If an hour or upwards has elapsed between the time a man has swallowed a poison and he is seen, it will be useless to cause vomiting. All that then can be done is to give milk to drink, or sweet oil, or soap and water, or white of eggs, if they can be got. The further treatment for particular kinds of poisons can only be followed out in hospital.

PONCHO.—The American soldiers during the war in that country made extensive use of the poncho, finding it to act the double purpose of cloak and *tente abri.* It may also be used as a sheet. It consists simply of a blanket or piece of waterproof cloth, with a slit in its middle through which the head may pass, and the *poncho* be thus worn in rainy weather. For campaigning purposes it is in many respects better suited than the ordinary *tente abri,* as a man may make himself warm with it in bivouac. Officers can and ought to provide themselves with a poncho whenever ordered on service or to *autumn manœuvres.*

PRECAUTIONS AGAINST DISEASE.—The soldier should know that however much may be done by his medical officers to suggest measures for the preservation of the health of *the whole* regiment, yet those measures will not be effectual with individuals unless each one takes the necessary care of his own health, and avoids the obvious causes of disease by which he may be surrounded. In hot countries, where the CLIMATE alone weakens the strength, avoid adding to the exhaustion by unnecessary or violent exertion. The morning and evening are the proper times for exercise in such places ; but during the heat of the day, instead of spending the whole time in sleep, the body should be kept moderately active, either in games or recreations now so abundantly provided within barracks. To remain all day in a close barrack-room with a number of perspiring comrades is most injurious to health, and has been the cause in former days of a great deal of pulmonary consumption as well as of other diseases. Excesses in and errors of diet are to be avoided; so also is the use of unwholesome or tainted meats, fish, shell-fish, &c. See that you avoid sleeping in cellars or underground apartments ; that you have free ventilation. Be careful with regard to clothing, wearing woollen whenever the climate is damp or "chilly." Drink coffee instead of spirits or beer, or, in very hot weather, use lime-juice and water to quench thirst. If you feel out of sorts, moderate the quantity of food usually taken, but do not delay to seek medical advice. As it is necessary to be up early to obtain the fresh air, so a siesta or short mid-day sleep is needed to enable a person to be out of bed at *gun-fire.* Excesses in drink, or, in fact, any abuse, sooner or later destroy health ; they should, therefore, be most carefully avoided. When particular forms of disease are prevalent, men should guard against them as much as possible, living with the greatest care, avoiding dissipation of all kinds, and, as far as may be

possible, having cheerful occupations in their leisure hours.
—*See* HEALTH, HYGIENE, &c.

PRICKLY HEAT.—This is a source of great suffering to
many soldiers in India, especially the stout and first
arrivals.   It is most frequent during the rainy season,
causing such a degree of itching and *pricking* of the skin
as sometimes to interfere with sleep.   The only measures
that a soldier can take to guard against the affection include
light clothing, abstinence from *heating* food, moderation in
drink, and *quiet*, in so far as he can indulge in the latter.
The use of *flour* as powder on the affected part relieves
the itching.   The use of the nails should be absolutely
resisted.

QUININE.—This medicine is extensively used in the army
in the treatment of ague, as well as for its prevention.   For
the latter purpose, it is issued as a regular ration in some
unhealthy countries and districts.   In Hong Kong, on the
coast of Africa, and at some Indian stations it is so, more
especially at Peshawur, great confidence being placed in
its efficacy for this purpose by medical officers.   The usual
form in which it is given is that of quinine wine.—*See*
AGUE, MALARIA, &c.

RAILWAY CARRIAGES.—Those on the broad gauge will
carry 5 soldiers with arms on a seat, or from 50 to 60 per
carriage; those on the narrow gauge 4 on a seat, or 32 per
carriage.   An American first-class car will carry 40.   It
is usual on some railways to allot carriages for 10 passengers to 8 soldiers only; those for 8 passengers to 6 soldiers.
Railway carriages are now used extensively for the con-
veyance of sick and wounded, but require to be specially
fitted up for the purpose, as they are in America and in
Germany.   During the Franco-Prussian war, the means
and organization for conveying troops by rail attained a
perfection hitherto unknown.   Every arrangement was
made at stations for supplying them with food and all

requirements, and elaborate instructions issued for the guidance of officers and men concerned:

RATIONS.—The following are the scales of rations, per man, allowed under the various conditions named, viz. :—

In the Field.—Bread 1½ lb., or biscuit 1 lb., fresh or salt meat 1 lb., coffee ⅓ oz., tea ⅛ oz., sugar 2 oz., salt ½ oz., pepper $\frac{1}{36}$ oz.

In Quarters.—Bread 1 lb., fresh meat with bone 12 oz., supplemented by extra messing.—*See* FOOD.

On Expeditions.—Various additions are made to the rations on the recommendation of the P. M. O. The meat ration is sometimes increased to 1½ lb., and compressed or fresh vegetables given, 2 oz. of the former or 8 oz. of the latter, or lime juice 1 oz. daily, when neither can be obtained.

In India.—The daily ration consists of 1 lb. of bread, 1 lb. of beef or mutton, 1 lb. of potatoes or other vegetables, 4 oz. of rice, ⅔ oz. of salt, $\frac{5}{7}$ oz. of tea, 1$\frac{3}{7}$ oz. of coffee, and 2 oz. of sugar.

On board Ship.—The scale of rations allows a variety, according to each day of the week, thus :—

Sunday.—12 oz. preserved meat, 1 lb. fresh bread, 1 pint porter, 2 oz. preserved potatoes, 2 oz. sugar, ½ oz. tea.

Monday.—12 oz. salt beef, 6 oz. flour, 1 oz. suet, 2 oz. raisins, 1 oz. compressed mixed vegetables, 12 oz. biscuit, 1 pint porter, 4 oz. sugar, ½ oz. tea.

Tuesday.—12 oz. preserved meat, 1 lb. fresh bread, 4 oz. rice, 1 pint porter, 2 oz. sugar, ½ oz. tea.

Wednesday.—12 oz. salt pork, $\frac{2}{9}$ pint split peas, 1 oz. compressed vegetables, 12 oz. biscuit, 1 pint porter, 2 oz. sugar, ½ oz. tea.

Thursday.—12 oz. salt beef, 6 oz. flour, 1 oz. suet, 2 oz. raisins, 1 oz. compressed vegetables, 1 lb. fresh bread, 1 pint porter, 4 oz. sugar, ½ oz. tea.

Friday.—12 oz. preserved meat, 12 oz. biscuit, 1 pint porter, 2 oz. preserved potatoes, 2 oz. sugar, ½ oz. tea.

Saturday.—12 oz. salt pork, $\frac{2}{9}$ pint peas, 1 oz. compressed vegetables, 1 lb. fresh bread, 1 pint porter, 2 oz. sugar, $\frac{1}{2}$ oz. tea.

Weekly.—$\frac{1}{8}$ pint vinegar, $\frac{1}{2}$ oz. mustard, 6 oz. pickles, $\frac{1}{6}$ oz. pepper. 2 oz. salt.

Spirits on board ship are now issued only on the certificate of the medical officer in charge.

Lime juice is issued on the recommendation of the surgeon ; an allowance of sugar being given at the same time.

Autumn Manœuvres.—The daily ration of provisions and groceries will be as follows, the men being subject to the usual stoppages, viz. :—

Ordinary Rations : 1 lb. of bread or 1 lb. of biscuit; 1 lb. meat, fresh or salt. *Extra issue :* $\frac{1}{4}$ lb. of cheese, when deemed necessary and ordered by officers commanding divisions, for men on outlying pickets and in situations where difficulties exist in issuing the ordinary ration. *Groceries :* $\frac{1}{4}$ lb. bread, $\frac{1}{3}$ oz. tea, 2 oz. sugar, $\frac{1}{2}$ oz. $\frac{1}{36}$ oz. pepper.

The scale of rations given to the men of the *Red River Expedition* was a very good one. It consisted of the following, viz. :—1 lb. of salt pork, or 1$\frac{1}{2}$ lbs. fresh meat ; 1 lb. of biscuits, or 1$\frac{1}{2}$ lb. of fresh bread ; $\frac{1}{3}$ pint of beans, or $\frac{1}{4}$ lb. of preserved potatoes; 1 oz. of tea, 2 oz of sugar, $\frac{1}{2}$ oz. of salt, when fresh meat is issued, $\frac{1}{36}$ oz. of pepper.— *See* FOOD.

RECRUITS.—Although every possible care is taken in the selection of healthy young men as recruits, the fact is undeniable that large numbers break down in health during their training. The more delicate among them, and those who had been poorly fed prior to enlistment, should be treated more tenderly, as regards duty and *gymnastics*, than the strong and stout. Non-commissioned officers should encourage them to spend their surplus money in the purchase of wholesome articles of food. They should be permitted as much and as long continuous sleep and rest as are practicable. When at drill or exercise the clothing, especially the tunic at the neck and breast should fit loosely or be open. The waist belt of the trousers should also be loose; otherwise young men are liable to become ruptured while undergoing drill. The future moral career of recruits often depends upon the discretion and tact shown by non-commissioned officers towards them; and inasmuch as physical health or disease are often direct results of a man's own conduct, the bearing of this subject on hygiene must be manifest.

REST.—Absolute rest and quiet is one of the most valuable aids to medical treatment of sickness, and is indispensable in that of wounds and injuries. It is equally important where great fatigue or exposure has been undergone; if indulged in for a little the effects of both are soon recovered from, while if not practicable, or not taken advantage of, illness of some kind, most probably fever of a low type will be induced, and perhaps the life of the person endangered. After fatigue spirits or stimulants do no good whatever. What is required is *rest*, and, it may be, a little extra food, to make up for the waste of tissue.

RINGWORM.—The affection commonly known by this name is of very frequent occurrence in India, attacking the "fork" and inner part of the thighs, and often causing great discomfort. It is believed to be more frequent among stout persons than among those of more spare habit. The best means of guarding against it seems to be care in keeping the parts as dry as possible, and being careful to wearing clean clothes. The application of the juice of a fresh lemon is a popular remedy in India, and probably of use when employed early in the disease. The affection once set in extends and becomes more obstinate the longer it is left untouched.

RUPTURE, OR HERNIA.—The general cause of this accident is violent exertion, as that of raising a weight, pumping, &c. The occurrence is generally made known by a feeling as if something had given way in the groin, followed by a soft swelling sooner or later. The best thing in such a case to be done is to lay the patient on his back, and then by a little gentle handling the rupture usually disappears with a gurgle. At the earliest opportunity the man should consult the surgeon, who will apply for a truss. If at any time the rupture should come down and not admit of being readily put back, let the patient be placed upon a stretcher and carried to hospital. Delay for a few hours in such a case may render a dangerous operation necessary.

Scurvy.—The disease properly called scurvy is attended by bleeding from the gums, blotches of a blue colour on the legs, great weakness, and in extreme cases death. It was formerly common on board ship. It is now comparatively rare, but may take place not only at sea, but on shore, from great fatigue, exposure, and bad or insufficient food, or sameness in diet. Its best preventive is the opposite of the conditions just mentioned—that is, good, plenty, and variety in food, cleanliness, good accommodation. Juicy vegetables and fruit prevent and cure it. Wine and beer are also good for either purpose. Fresh meat, pickles, new potatoes, and vinegar are also good. The Esquimaux give *raw fresh* meat as a remedy for scurvy, and this method of treatment was used with success during the siege of Paris, when vegetables, fruit, pickles, or lime juice were all alike unobtainable.

Sea Kit.—The following are the orders in force on the subject of soldiers' kits for sea voyages—viz. :—

I.—FOR THE MAURITIUS, CEYLON, STRAITS SETTLEMENTS, CHINA, AND INDIA (IF *via* THE CAPE OF GOOD HOPE).

Frocks, blue serge	1
Trousers, blue serge, without stripes, pair	1
Neckerchief, cotton	1
Soap, marine, pieces	8

Soap, yellow	4
Pipe-clay, balls	3
Blacking, tins of	2
Brush, scrubbing	1
Knife, clasp	1
Bag	1
Needles and thread. set	1
Tobacco, lbs.	3
Cap, blue worsted	1

Shirts (in addition to kit) { check ... ... 2 / or / flannel 1

Belts, flannel	2

(Not required when flannel shirts are worn.)

II.—FOR INDIA (IF *via* EGYPT).

Frock, white drill	1
Trousers, ditto, pair	1
Soap, marine, pieces	4
Soap, yellow	4
Pipe-clay, ball...	1
Blacking, tin of	1
Brush, scrubbing	1
Knife, clasp	1
Bag	1
Needles and thread, set	1
Tobacco, lb.	$1\frac{1}{2}$
Cap, blue worsted	1
Water-bottle	1
Belts, flannel	1

(For further particulars see Horse Guards General Order 76, October 1867).

III.—FOR AUSTRALIA, TASMANIA, AND NEW ZEALAND.

Frocks, blue serge	1
Trousers, blue serge, without stripes, pair	1
Neckerchief, cotton	1
Socks, worsted (in addition to kit), pair	1
Boots, knee, pair	1
Soap, marine, pieces	12
Soap, yellow	4
Pipe-clay, balls	3

Shirts (in addition to kit) { check ... ... 2 / or / flannel 1

Brush, scrubbing	1

Blacking, tins of	...	...	...	...	...	2
Knife, clasp	...	...	...	...	...	1
Needles and thread, set	...	...	...	...	1
Tobacco, lbs. ...	...	...	...	...	...	3
Bag, in lieu of havresack	...	...	...	...	1
Cap, blue worsted	...	...	...	...	...	1

IV.—FOR THE CAPE OF GOOD HOPE.

Frock, blue serge	...	...	...	...	...	1
Trousers, blue serge, without stripes	...	...	1
Bag, in lieu of havresack	...	...	...	...	1
Soap, marine, pieces ...	...	...	...	...	4
Soap, yellow ...	...	...	...	...	...	2
Needles and thread, set	...	...	...	...	1
Pipe-clay, ball ...	...	...	...	...	...	1
Tobacco, lb. ...	...	...	...	...	...	$1\frac{1}{2}$
Cap, blue worsted	...	...	...	...	...	1

V.—FOR THE WEST INDIES, CANADA, AND ST. HELENA.

Frock, blue serge	...	...	...	...	...	1
Trousers, blue serge, without stripes, pair ...	...	1
Bag, in lieu of havresack	...	...	...	...	1

SERVICE.—A soldier ordered on service should, as far as in his power, be provided with new articles of clothing. He should take nothing with him that is old. His boots and socks should be well fitting, the latter warm. His *housewife* should be well supplied. He should have with him a strong pocket-knife, provide himself with a small bottle of salt and pepper for seasoning his food, as also a toothbrush, the use of which he will find very refreshing. His officers of course provide for his larger wants which are supplied in accordance with "Regulations."

In order that the soldier may be enabled to withstand the fatigues of service and carry the weight of kit, arms, and accoutrements he must be well fed, and amply clothed. It is the duty of officers to see that the men are well housed, that they have means of amusement and of diverting their minds from the inevitable trials and discomforts of war. Before going on "duty," the soldier should have a hot meal, either solid or consisting of coffee and bread as the case may be. They will now find the advantage of each man being able to cook for himself. Of course the responsible officers will see that their men are not more fatigued or harassed than circumstances of the service render absolutely necessary, and experience has shown the impropriety of sending the same men into battle on two successive days, unless they have been brilliantly successful in the first. Among the instructions laid down for men on service are the following. Avoid irregularities, learn to mend your own clothes, and even boots, keep your hair short, preserve cleanliness of clothes and person as much as possible, washing the whole body as often as you can ; avoid as far as possible exposing yourself to the causes of diseases incidental to service, be careful as far as possible that boots, socks, and clothing are in good order. Further good advice is that given to the French soldier, namely, to cook from time to time whatever food he may have in his mess-tin, or if he has not time for that, to grill a little meat if he can ; to have as a small reserve store with him from day to day, as a little cooked meat, a little bread or biscuit, salt, and pepper. If he can carry a small tin of preserved meat, or meat essence, he may always be able to prepare for himself, a *savoury*, if not very nutritive meal.

SHIP, ON BOARD OF.—The general regulations of the army contain instructions for the good of the mass on board, and individuals should endeavour to give effect in their own persons to the spirit of those instructions, remembering how very fearful a thing it is when an outbreak of sickness takes place while a vessel is far away at sea. Cleanliness and free ventilation " below " are the great safeguards to be observed. Disinfectants are recommended to be used, but they prove no sufficient substitutes for cleanliness of the ship and cleanliness of each individual on board. In a hot climate no harm whatever need be feared from sleeping near a windsail or a hatchway. Draughts of air are then both grateful and beneficial. When, however, men sleep on deck and *not* under an awning they expose themselves to be attacked by various diseases, as dysentery, rheumatism, moon blindness, &c. They should spend as much of their time as possible on deck, indulging in such exercises and amusements as they can. Better for them to get an occasional wetting, with plenty of exercise, than to be dry and lazy. During *washing decks* in the morning men should freely *souse* themselves, so long as the weather admits of it. As preventives against scurvy, they should use all the vinegar, pickles, and lime juice they can get.

It is injurious for men in a state of perspiration to rush on deck insufficiently clothed, and thus expose themselves to the draughts of wind, or it may be rain; so also it is for a man to fall asleep under such circumstances. Although free ventilation "below" is desirable, yet the mouths of windsails ought to open at a level *under* the cot in which a man may "swing." It is at all times desirable to keep the lower deck as dry as possible, and to avoid having any wet clothes below. A man if obliged at night to go on deck, should be careful to dress himself sufficiently, for however short a time it may be. On arriving at foreign ports the greatest care is necessary in regard to meat, fish, and fruit offered for sale by natives. Pork and fish, are as a rule, very dangerous under such circumstances, and ought to be avoided. Cleanliness of clothing and person is necessary, and must be carefully attended to. A man sick on board ship requires every consideration to be shown him. Under the most favourable circumstances he cannot possibly have all the comforts obtainable on shore.

SHIRTS.—Perhaps for all purposes, and having regard to the life and work of a soldier, woollen shirts are preferable to others. In cold weather or climates there is no question on the subject. In hot, they are also best suited for preventing sudden chills after severe exertion; but then their material should be of light quality. Occasionally men are met with whose skin is so tender that *flannel* is absolutely unbearable. In this respect, and the difficulty of washing it properly, this material is not suited for general wear by the soldier; but there are more than one kind of substance, partly composed of wool and partly of cotton, that are in all respects suited for wear when the thicker and coarser could perhaps not be borne next to the skin.—*See* CLOTHING.

SICK.—The proportion of sick to strength usually looked for varies much according to condition and circumstances. In the United Kingdom hospital arrangements are made for 6 per cent. effectives; in India, for 10, 12, or more, according to station; on the ordinary march, 5; on service, 10. There are conditions under which these ratios are far exceeded, as during epidemics, and at some notoriously unhealthy stations. The fact may be mentioned, however, that it by no means follows that a high rate of *sickness* is attended by a high rate of mortality. The reverse is sometimes the case.

SICKNESS.—No man when attacked with sickness should delay an hour in seeking relief. In many instances a fatal, or at any rate, severe, attack may be warded off by timely medical aid. It is a delusion to believe that real illness can either be *shaken off* or *fought against*. It is but an indication of our common mortality, and no man can either shake off or fight against mortality. Immediately a soldier becomes sick he should be removed from the barrack-room and sent to hospital, this as much for his own well-being as for the comfort of his comrades.—*See* DISEASE, ILLNESS, &c.

Sickness on Service.—Soldiers should know that on service sickness causes more inefficiency and more deaths than occur by battle; and in order to avoid the chances of being themselves struck down it is well that they should know its principal causes. The forms of disease most prevalent during time of war are *typhoid* and *typhus fever* and *dysentery*. Among their most prominent causes are bad food, over-crowding, fatigue, and exposure to the weather.

The object of military *hygiene* is to indicate the means by which these influences may be counteracted; and it behoves individual men to fully observe the regulations laid down from time to time with this object, knowing that if once they become attacked by illness, their recovery is, under such circumstances, at all times a matter of distant uncertainty.

SKIN DISEASES.—The extent to which these prevail in the army is now small compared to what was formerly the case, the improvement being chiefly due to the greater care now paid to cleanliness of the person. They are by no means extinct however, but are best guarded against by cleanliness of person and of clothing, avoiding the use of woollen soiled with perspiration or otherwise, avoiding intercourse with persons of dirty habits in public-houses or other places of common resort, never washing or bathing in water that has already been used, or drying the face or body with a towel already soiled. Some of these affections are very catching, and all are more or less difficult of cure unless treated very early in their attack.

SLEEP.—A soldier ought to have eight hours sleep out of every twenty-four. This becomes of course impossible when he is on guard, but should as far as circumstances allow, be made up for afterwards. The requirements of the service and consideration for the health of the men as a body render it necessary that they keep early hours. In India, however, as a regular thing, and the practice is allowed in some regiments at home, the men are permitted to make down their beds after dinner for an hour, a measure not only for their comfort, but for their health. On the line of march, as it is necessary to be up early, so men should go to sleep early. Men should not be unnecessarily *roused* out of their sleep; hence any noise or *larking* in the barrack-room at night ought to be checked. There is of course a difference between a man having the quantity of sleep that is necessary for health, and being "heavy headed."

A good soldier must necessarily be an active man. Before going to sleep at night, health and comfort alike require that a man should undress, and put on a different shirt from that worn during the day.

SNAKE BITE.—The means recommended to be taken in the case of bite by a poisonous snake is to cut or *burn* the part immediately ; the latter is perhaps the preferable plan. A ligature or handkerchief to be tied as tightly as possible around the bitten limb between the part bitten and the trunk of the body. The person to have plenty of spirits given to him, and if possible kept walking. If the snake be really poisonous, and of large size, the case will as a rule be desperate indeed.—*See* BITES.

SOAP.—So much of personal comfort depends upon a soldier being provided with soap, that he should, under all circumstances take care to have a piece readily available. On service he should carry it in his havresack, remembering that the late General Sir C. Napier considered this article to be of such prime necessity that, according to him, all a soldier needed in the shape of kit was "two towels and a piece of soap." There often happen occasions when, from one cause or another, it is impossible to obtain soap, as during some military expeditions. Under such circumstances, bran, oatmeal, peasmeal, clay, more especially fuller's earth, may be used as substitutes. In fact, in India the natives find the mud of the Ganges serves all the purposes of soap. The ashes of many plants, if boiled or mixed with water, yield an alkali which, for washing clothes, may be used in place of soap, and there are several plants met with in foreign countries which, when bruised and mixed with water, form a *lather*, having all the properties of that from ordinary soap. If a man wishes to wash his person thoroughly and has no soap with him, he had best smear himself well with mud, and then proceed as if he were taking his bath in the ordinary way. Fancy soaps are coloured by various chemical substances that are injurious to the skin ; hence the best kinds for general use are the white and yellow. In India the *soap berry* is used by the natives, and serves all the purposes of the article whence it takes its name.

SOCKS.—For all purposes, woollen socks are better than cotton for use by the soldier, notwithstanding that they render the feet soft on the march, by their warmth, and cause blisters unless they fit well and are in good repair. Men should be careful when selecting their socks that their size is suited to the foot, and when holes occur in them, the darning should be carefully done, otherwise the part that is mended will irritate the foot. Foreign soldiers use socks very little. The Germans use a long bandage of linen instead. Practice enables them to apply it so neatly that it supports the foot without irritating it. On the march and active service it is easily kept clean and readily washed. Pieces of linen or cotton cloth may also be used as substitutes for socks. These should be a foot square, be washed every day, and smeared with tallow. If put on neatly they will stand a march without a wrinkle taking place in them. To put them on, the foot is placed on one of the diagonals, the triangles on the right and left are then folded over, then the triangle in front of the toes, and with a little practice these can be so arranged as to be without a wrinkle. The use of socks that are soiled "soften" the feet ; if full of holes, they cause blisters, and, moreover, only insufficiently protect the feet. When they have become wet, they ought to be changed with the least pos·sible delay.—*See* CLOTHING.

SPACE.—According to Regulations, soldiers are allowed space at the rate of 600 cubic feet in barracks, and 400 in huts. On the march, a cavalry soldier occupies one yard, an infantry man 2 feet, irrespective of the space between troops, companies, and regiments ; in hospitals, the cubic space allowed is 1,000 to 1,500 feet, according to climate, with 80 to 100 superficial feet. On board ship, 52 cubic

G

and 10½ superficial feet. The necessity of ample *space* is very nearly as great when troops are on the march or camp as when they are in barracks. The occurrence of *heat apoplexy* among those in India is found to be more frequent when marching in close column than when in open order. Epidemics also spread among crowds at places of pilgrimage quite as much as among those in barracks or towns.— *See* ACCOMMODATION.

SPIRITS.—The action of spirits upon the stomach is literally to *dry* up its tissues and check the secretion of its natural juices upon which digestion depends. Hence it is that a man who is addicted to spirit drinking is unable to take proper food, or to digest it when he has taken it. A good many years ago the surgeon of a regiment in India, where spirit-drinking prevailed to a fearful extent, invited the men to come with him to the *dead-house*, and see for themselves in the stomachs of those who died, the effects of spirits, and it is said that the measure did more than all others that had been taken to check the vice. Under some conditions, such as cold or wet, a *small* dram may for a time be *grateful*, but that even then it is unnecessary and injurious in the long run has been proved by late experience. Thus, men exposed in the outposts around Paris during winter found in practice that the use of spirits really rendered them more sensitive to cold than they were before, and many accordingly abandoned them for *coffee*. It has also been found that in ordinary marches men who are habitual spirit-drinkers are unable to stand fatigue so well as the more temperate, and that in hot countries such as India, the very great majority of cases of *Heat* APOPLEXY that prove fatal occur in confirmed spirit-drinkers. Medical men know well that the practice of taking *nips* to prevent *cholera, dysentery*, and other diseases affecting the bowels, have in reality no such property unless they contain spices and other medical remedies, and when the latter are taken, they should be so as *tinctures*, under the prescription of the medical officer, instead of really furnishing an excuse for indulgence in strong drink. Another excuse for taking spirits is that a man needs a a dram of *bitters* to stay his stomach. A healthy stomach needs no bitters, and if deranged, the chances in the person of a soldier are that it is so from indulgence in spirits, in which case bitters will by no means improve it. Fortunately spirits are no longer obtainable in canteens. They were abolished in the American army ; in the Mutiny campaign men marched during the hot season best without them ; hence they may be disused in our army with the very best results to the soldiers both as regards health and character. In some foreign countries, especially in the Mediterranean, India, and China, various kinds of *spirits* are sold to soldiers by native vendors, the effects of which are maddening, and most injurious to health. For special exceptions see FOOD and MALARIA.

SPRAINS.—These are but the first stage of DISLOCATIONS. They may be caused by a false step, a twist, a fall, &c. Their actual nature consists of a stretching or twisting of the ligaments which retain the joints in their shape and strength. They are often very painful, and followed by great swelling of the parts. They sometimes render the person suffering from them unfit for duty for weeks, and by no means seldom unfit him altogether to remain in the army, more especially when the knee or ankle is the part affected. The first thing to be done is to lay the person in such a position that his weight is taken off the injured part. Cold water or spirits and water should be applied, and then the man carried to hospital. Soldiers should know that unless they remain quiet while under treatment in hospital for sprains of the ankle and knee, obstinate or incurable disease often results from their own indiscretion.

STABLES.—Such places should be carefully avoided by soldiers on service. They are said to have been used as temporary sleeping places during the American war, and they were so during the Franco-German, but with sufficiently unfavourable results to show how necessary it is to avoid similar dangers in future. Cases of GLANDERS occurred among the troops who had used them, those attacked by this terrible disease dying most miserably.

STARVATION BY HUNGER.—A strong man will not actually die from starvation in less than eight to ten days. If, therefore, a soldier should be accidentally left in such a position, he should bear this in mind, and surely help of some kind will reach him in that time. When help does come it must be carefully applied. Stimulants must be avoided, milk given—at first in small quantities, the person placed if possible in a bed, but not near the fire; then food given by little and little.

STINGS, whether by wasp or scorpion, are conveniently treated by applying to them the oil scooped out of a tobacco-pipe. Spirits, whether brandy or rum, may also be applied. If a soldier can obtain a little powder of ipecacuhana, its application to the part is a ready and effective cure. Hartshorn or *Eau de luce* is also excellent. Honey or sugar is said to be good as a remedy.

STRANGULATION, whether arising from HANGING or not, as in attempts at suicide, should be treated like DROWNING, with the addition that a little cold water, or spirits and water, should, from time to time, be dashed upon the face and chest.

STRAW.—If waterproof sheets are not issued in *camp,* straw for bedding will be given for troops halted for any considerable time, at the rate of 72 lbs. per 5 men, or 216 lbs. per bell tent. Half the quantity will be given to replace one-third portion at the end of 8 days, a complete change being made at the end of 24. Straw readily accumulates dirt and insects, and becomes offensive. It should therefore be taken outside the tent as often as possible, shaken, and aired. The men should avoid the filthy habit of spitting upon their camp straw. The French soldiers readily make their straw into mats by means of some string. This is preferable to loose straw, as they can often be hung up in the sun and beaten clean every day. —*See* CAMP.

STRETCHERS, called also BRANCARDS. — In placing a wounded or injured man upon a stretcher, care and tenderness in handling him are very necessary. *Stretcher-bearers* are regularly taught how to perform this duty, but regularly trained men are not under all circumstances available. The stretcher being placed on the ground alongside the injured man, so as to do away with the necessity of disturbing him, as far as possible, the first care should be to gently support any limb that may be broken, so as to prevent it from dangling or being painfully moved. Besides the man or men required to support the injured limb, two are required to move a man comfortably on to a stretcher. One of these stands over the patient in such a way that he can get his arms well round his body, locking his fingers behind ; the other does precisely the same thing round his hips. If the injured man can raise his arms so as to clasp the neck of him who stands in front, so much the better. Any how, the two supporters having got themselves into position to give them *purchase*, they should both together raise the patient, at the same time moving in unison, so as to lift him directly over the stretcher. He should then be lowered very gently upon it, something placed under his head, his position rendered as comfortable as it can be, and then removed to hospital.—*See* CARRYING. *See also* FRACTURES. Another convenient plan is to place the stretcher lengthways at the feet of the patient. A man places himself at either side, so as to get one arm well under the shoulders, the other under the hips, and having done so, clasps the hand of the one opposite. The third bearer takes care of the injured limb, and thus the patient is gently raised and slipped on the brancard.

SUN, EXPOSURE TO.—Although there are men who do not appear to suffer from exposure to the fiercest rays of an Indian sun, the rule decidedly is, among soldiers, that such exposure is extremely injurious, and often followed by fatal results. If under the influence of spirits, beer, or other intoxicating liquor, they are especially liable to suffer from exposure; therefore, the regulations are very properly framed with a view to discourage the practice of soldiers being out of doors while the power of the sun is great.

SUNSTROKE.—*See also* HEAT APOPLEXY.—This is not uncommon among soldiers when marching during very hot weather. It chiefly occurs, however, among those who have indulged much beforehand in spirits or beer, being rare indeed among the absolutely sober. In India it has been found to take place when troops march in close column more than it does when they are in open order. Its signs are, the man becoming insensible, the face deadly pale or red, and *suffused;* the head and body intensely hot; the eyes red, and turned up; the breathing, at first rapid, afterwards slow and stertorous or snoring. The face and limbs are sometimes convulsed. The first thing to be done is to loosen the clothes, take off the pack, place the man in a comfortable position upon the ground in an open space, so that plenty of fresh air may reach him. Throw plenty of cold water upon the head and body. If a bottle of smelling salts is obtainable, place it, from time to time, under the nostrils, and send for a medical officer. To prevent it the best means are temperance, and during necessary exposure to keep the head and body moist by occasionally sponging, or throwing cold water over them..

SUSPENSORS.—The use of these articles, or *suspensory bandages* as they are sometimes called, is for a mounted soldier almost an actual necessity. Certainly every such man should use one, and there are many in the unmounted branches, especially while serving in hot climates, who do use them; whenever they are used, benefit will also be obtained from bathing *the parts* requiring them, with as cold water as is procurable.—*See* DRAGOONS.

SWIMMING.—Is not only an agreeable exercise, but it strengthens the constitution, gives power to the muscles, and developes the chest. A good swimmer may have it in his power to save a comrade, and thus earn a reward for a daring action. Men, however, until able to swim should bathe in company with some who can do so, and themselves avoid being foolhardy in so dangerous an element as water. In the course of military operations soldiers have often to swim across rivers or canals. When this is attempted, each should use a float of some kind, as a piece of wood, a bunch of reeds, or even corked bottles, or cooking vessels, any of which placed under the chest will be of material assistance to him. If under such circumstances a man is utterly unable to swim, floats should be placed under his arms and lashed firmly to him; he must then be *towed* across. For short distances, and provided the man who is unable to swim has sufficient confidence, he may simply place a hand upon each hip of a comrade who is able to swim well, and thus be guided across. A kind of float may also be made of a piece of intestine inflated and tied by a string at intervals, so as to make a swimming belt, by being placed around the chest under the armpits.

For a cavalry soldier to swim his horse and himself across a stream the best way is after getting into the stream for each man to hold on by the mane or tail of the horse, splashing water in the face of the animal with the free hand so as to guide him; of course, such a necessity is now-a-days of very rare occurrence, yet it may arise again as it has often done before. *The Queen's Regulations* direct that swimming shall be taught as a military duty, and that a list of swimmers shall be kept in each company, to give aid if need be on the occasion of bathing parades.

SWORDS, CUTS BY.—Bring the sides of the wound together with both hands and keep them in that position,

covering the part with some folds of cloth soaked in cold
water. Place the wounded man in such a position that the
tendency of the wound to be stretched open will be least.
If the wound is near a large joint, as the knee, the lips
should be carefully held together until the arrival of a
surgeon.—*See* WOUNDS.

TEETH.—Neglect of the teeth, so often seen among soldiers, is not only most offensive to their neighbours, but
injurious to the men's own health. The breath suffers, the
teeth themselves rot and decay, and the health of the person
is impaired by the presence, week after week, of decomposing matters around the teeth. All men who value their
own health, cleanliness, and comfort—not to speak of their
personal appearance in the eyes of others—ought carefully
to brush their teeth at least twice a day, using on each
occasion a rough hard brush and toothpowder of some kind.
The harder the brush and the harder the brushing, the
better ultimately for the state of the gums and teeth.
When toothache occurs, the man should consult the surgeon. The best toothpowder for use by the soldier is
charcoal, or equal parts of charcoal and camphorated
chalk.

TEMPERAMENT.—Much of a man's character depends
upon his natural *temperament*. He may certainly be able,
by the exercise of self-command, to modify his character,
but when he does so it is often at the cost of pain and
suffering to himself that his friends and comrades little
know of. In dealing with soldiers, therefore, it would be
well were it always possible to take their natural *temperament* into account, and with this view the following sum-
mary is given, viz. :—

1. *Sanguine*, characterized by moderate plumpness of
person and firmness of flesh, hair red or light chestnut,
eyes blue, complexion florid, skin soft and thin, habits
active, countenance animated, passions excitable, mind
volatile and unsteady.

2. *Phlegmatic*, by roundish body, softness of muscles, fair hair, light blue or grey eyes, the functions of body and mind inactive and dull.

3. *Bilious*, by moderate fullness and much firmness of flesh, harshly expressed outlines of person, hair black, eyes and complexion dark, features strongly marked and decided ; much energy, both of body and mind.

4. *Nervous*, by small and spare frame, slender muscles, quick movements, pale countenance, delicate health, the whole system active, senses acute, thoughts quick, imagination lively.

5. *Melancholic*—allied to *Bilious*—characterized by calmness and serious tendency of mind, tenacity of purpose, and tendency to take a gloomy view of matters.

These characteristics are only very briefly stated; yet it must be evident that the manner of dealing with the subjects of the temperaments noted must and ought to be very different; that, for example, what would make little or no impression upon a *cold* phlegmatic person, would render desperate the man of *nervous* and sensitive disposition. In these respects their enumeration is considered within the intended sphere of this work. Medical men are aware that the subjects of particular temperaments are liable to particular forms of disease.—*See* FOOD.

TENTS.—The Franco-German war proved that a campaign may take place in Europe and the troops be unprovided with tents. The Germans used none; and the time taken up by the French in packing their *tentes abri* is believed in some instances to have been the cause of their defeat in particular actions. So in America, during the war of the Secession, tents were little, if at all, used. In hot countries, however, as India, during the greater part of the year, it would be death to the men were they to march without tents. The following are the tents in most general use :—

1. *Circular.* Used everywhere by our troops except in India. It is 10 ft. high, 12½ ft. in diameter at the base ;

the ropes extend 18 inches all round; it is made of canvas, consists of a velise, pole, bag containing 42 pins and 2 mallets, and weighs 74 lbs. It is supposed to contain 15 men.

2. *Tente abri* of the French, consists of 2 sheets, 2 poles, 7 pins ; weighs about 11 lbs., and holds 2 men.

3. *Bengal tent.* One to every 16 men.

4. *Bombay tents* hold 22 men each.

5. *Madras tents* hold 25 men each.

Hospital marquee is intended to accommodate 18 sick, but this number is really too great. It contains 3,336 feet of cubic air; weighs 512 lbs.

THIRST.—Soldiers should know that when fresh water is not to be had thirst may, for a time at least, be satisfied to some degree by bathing in salt water, a portion being thus absorbed by the skin. To prevent the risk of thirst on service, they should take a good drink before starting in the morning. It is also recommended, when marching in a hot and dry country, to place a cloth over the mouth. It is said that a small piece of fat put into the mouth from time to time has a similar effect. If fresh water is to be had, although in very small quantities, take a little, even if only a tea-spoonful, at intervals. This will stay great thirst for a time. The danger of taking large draughts of water or other liquid, to satisfy thirst on the march, is well known and ought to be avoided. One plan of quenching thirst with a small quantity of water is said to be to take a mouthful, and, without swallowing it, to breathe over it by the mouth, letting the breath escape by the nose, repeating this operation four or five times with each mouthful of water. The air thus moistened, passing over the fauces, relieves the feeling of thirst. The feeling of thirst is always greater in hot climates than in those that are temperate ; it is also increased after partaking of salted or highly seasoned food. In either case, small quantities of liquid, taken at short intervals, will be more likely to quench it than one or two large draughts.

THROAT, SORE.—A common affection, as a result of exposure to wet and cold. The best provisional treatment is to surround the neck with fomentations or poultice, to inhale the steam of hot water, and take hot drinks. To avoid the risk of attack, be careful that clothing, including stockings, be sufficiently warm. If wet, they should be changed without delay. The use of a gargle, made with a little vinegar and red pepper, sometimes has the effect of checking an attack of this kind.

TOBACCO.—Without being a necessity, and although when used to excess its effects are decidedly injurious to health, still there is no doubt that its moderate use supplies a want. that would be otherwise greatly felt by many soldiers. It moreover soothes and gives men enjoyment of which it would be very much to be regretted if they were to be deprived. It is often said that the practice of smoking tobacco prevents the smoker from being affected with *malaria*, and protects him against infection ; but there is really no proof that it does the one or the other. The immediate injury to health caused by tobacco in excess arises in the shape of disordered digestion, palpitation, *nervousness*, and a sense of *stupidity*.

TREES.—A grove of trees although perhaps good as shelter during a temporary halt in the heat of the day as in India, is objectionable for long occupation, and as a rule for *camp* or *bivouac* during a night. It acts as a shade from the sun, and as shelter from the rain, but is a source of risk in a storm, partly on account of the wind eddying round individual trees, partly from the liability of some to be thrown down, and partly from their liability to act as conductors of LIGHTNING in storms. All these considerations have no relation to the military advantages of trees, whether singly or in groves. No doubt, however, a grove of trees prevents intense heat or intense cold, and in either respect has its peculiar advantage. A belt of trees between barracks and a marsh acts as a barrier against *malaria*.

Also, trees in the vicinity, if not very close, are agreeable and wholesome in all climates.

URINE, RETENTION OF.—A man, probably has suffered from stricture, or indulges in a debauch. He finds himself unable to void his urine. He must at once prepare to be taken to hospital. In the meantime he may apply hot fomentations over the lower part of the belly. He should avoid taking drinks of any kinds, more especially spirits, as these by increasing the secretion of urine will materially add to the existing evil. The affection is a serious one, and will in all probability require the use of instruments.

VACCINATION.—The orders in regard to vaccinating all recruits who join, and the families of such as are married with leave are very strict. Soldiers should know, however, that to the care with which vaccination and re-vaccination are performed in the army we must attribute in a great measure the comparative rarity of small-pox in the army. Surgeons of regiments have greater means than most civil practitioners possess of obtaining pure vaccine matter, as they know the history of the parents of the children from whom it is usually taken, and the fact, of no case having yet occurred of *disease* being inoculated in vaccination from a soldier's child speaks for itself. It should be understood that vaccination does not altogether prevent the occurrence of small-pox. It diminishes the liability to attack and decreases the risks of death among persons attacked. The practice of re-vaccination is also compulsory in the army, and by way of pointing out to the soldier the good results that follow the operation, the following extract from a Report on the subject by the Directors of the Small-pox Hospital, at Hampstead, is appended.

" The necessity of re-vaccination when the protective power of the primary vaccination has to a great· extent passed away, cannot be too strongly urged. No greater argument to prove the efficacy of this precaution can be

adduced than the fact that out of upwards of 14,000 cases
received into the hospital, only four well-authenticated
cases were treated in which re-vaccination had been properly performed, and these were light attacks. Further
conclusive evidence is afforded by the fact that all the
nurses and servants of the hospital, to the number at one
time of upwards of 300, who are hourly brought into
the most intimate contact with the disease, who constantly
breathe its atmosphere, and than whom none can be more
exposed to its contagion, have, with but few exceptions,
enjoyed complete immunity from its attacks. These
exceptions were cases of nurses or servants whose re-
vaccination in the pressure of the epidemic was over-
looked, and who speedily took the disease; and one
case was that of a nurse, who, having had small-pox
previously, was not re-vaccinated, and took the disease a
second time."

VEGETABLES.—The use of vegetables as food is absolutely
necessary in order to keep the man in health, and when
either from our not taking them, or their not being procurable, the bodily system is deprived of them *scurvy* is the
result. In India where during some seasons they cannot
be procured, the Government authorises an issue of lime-
juice being made, and in this way averts the evils that
would otherwise arise. In some countries there are numbers of common weeds that can be used as substitutes for
ordinary vegetables. The French soldiers are adepts at dis-
covering such, and it would be an excellent thing if ours
were equally so. The most wholesome vegetables are potatoes, cabbages, and turnips; next to them carrots, parsnips,
&c. Many vegetables can be used cold, mixed with vinegar, as salad, and it is a pity that they are not more used
than they are by English soldiers.

VENEREAL DISEASES.—In whatever form these diseases
occur, recovery from them must always be looked upon as
uncertain. By their ulterior effects they embitter and

shorten the life of their subject, and in the event of his marrying may affect his wife and children, being transmitted from him. Concealment or delay in seeking treatment increases those risks. Treatment by quacks and such persons, as soldiers too often resort to in many cases, increase the evil results of the disease, hence the regimental medical officer ought always to be resorted to. Inasmuch as there is only one way in which the affections are contracted, so it becomes an easy matter, with the exercise of a little moderation, to avoid them. The excitement of a *spree* is certainly not worth its attendant risks.

VENTILATION.—If soldiers would but believe it, fresh air is the best, as it is the natural purifier of rooms rendered temporarily offensive by the presence of men. The ventilators provided in barrack-rooms are most serviceable in preserving health, provided they are in suitable working order. The practice of *stopping* them at night only injures the men themselves, by preventing the escape, it may be, of odours caused by the presence of one or more intoxicated men. When the troops quit their barracks for drill in the morning, the windows should be thrown completely open. It may be useful for the men to know that with their breath and perspiration very minute portions from their lungs and skin are thrown off ; these, if not removed by ventilation, cling to the walls and furniture, decay, and are inhaled again by the men in breathing. Thus they can understand how diseases, consumption, and others become propagated among them. Cold weather ought not to be made an excuse for the neglect of ventilation, whether of barracks, huts, or tents. The officers under such circumstances will apply for the issue of extra blankets. If a ventilator acts improperly so as to admit the draught or rain directly upon a person, the defect should be reported, so that the necessary alteration may be made. In pitching tents care is of course taken that sufficient distance exists between them to admit of free circulation of air among them. Grates and fire-places are efficient means of ventilation in rooms ; hence the latter should be left open when fires are discontinued.—*See* AIR, BARRACKS, &c.

VOMITING may arise from violent exertion, a chill, great annoyance, improper or too much food, from what is commonly called a *bilious* attack, and so on. It may also take place as the commencement of a severe illness or fever, and during the prevalence of CHOLERA may be itself the first sign of the person being seized with that disease.

In order to give temporary relief to the person attacked, undo his clothes, after the first great effort, give him a little warm tea or cold water. Either of these is preferable to spirits and water. If the vomiting persists, apply a hot brick or bottle to the stomach, while arrangements are being made to send the man to hospital. Of course, care will be taken when applying the brick that it be wrapped in a blanket or some other woollen cloth, so as to prevent it from coming directly in contact with the skin, and perhaps burning it.

WATER.—That for drinking or cooking purposes should be fresh and clear. That obtained from wells or springs is the purest, and in an enemy's country that from the latter source should be used if obtainable, as it is least likely to contain impurities. That from the middle of a stream is purer and better than such as is got from near the sides ; that from marshes and ditches should be avoided. Where stagnant water *must* be used, a piece of bread thrown into it and allowed to remain for a few minutes, removes in some degree its bad qualities. If muddy, it should be passed through a flannel or linen cloth, or through a handkerchief. It may also be purified by being passed through a bed of sand and charcoal some inches thick, by putting a little alum and charcoal in it, or by the use of the nut used by the natives for that purpose (*Strychnos ptatorum*). In many parts of India, wells and tanks furnish the only means of water supply. The French add a little vinegar or spirits to the water of inferior quality, and believe that in

some degree these arrest its bad qualities; it is considered
in England, however, that they do not. No man should
start on a march without his water-bottle being full, and
he should further avoid the risk of thirst by taking some
liquid at the same time, whether as tea, coffee, or water.
It is considered that in the course of a day in a hot
country two quarts of water is the smallest quantity a man
drinks.

The allowance of water for all purposes in barracks is
as follows, viz. : officers and men at the rate of 12 gallons
per head; women, 12 gallons; children, 4 gallons. Horses,
in the cavalry, 8 gallons ; in artillery and military train,
10 gallons. At sea, the common allowance is, 6 pints, per
head, on board ship, while out of the tropics ; 1 gallon in
the tropics. For horses, 8 gallons each.

Troops on the line of march should carefully avoid drinking water directly from streams or brooks. Leeches and
other noxious creatures and things are not unfrequently
taken into the mouth or get into the nostrils. The presence
of a leech may cause weeks of suffering, leading to ill-
health. The water should always be drank from a vessel,
or in the absence of one, taken up in the hands, or filtered
through a handkerchief.

WATERPROOF —The use of a waterproof sheet between a
man's person and the ground in the bivouac, is unquestion-
ably beneficial. So, of course, would one be over him
under such circumstances, provided the climate or season is
temperate. The former would equally be useful in a hot
climate, but then the latter would be unbearable. The
good health of the troops during the American war was in
a great part attributed to the use by them of waterproof
sheets and cloaks. The French troops in Algeria are said
to have suffered from rheumatism from wearing them,
as while the rain was kept out the perspiration was kept
from evaporating, and so, liability to a chill induced. On
the West Coast of Africa waterproof clothing was not used,
at any rate when I was there, but instead of it, Europeans

wore suits of thick blanketing when likely to be exposed
to rain. When this kind of material is used, the flexible
description is preferable to the more resisting. A sheet,
say 7 feet by 4, with eyelets along one side can by means
of a cord run through them be converted into a cape when
required.

To render cloth waterproof, rub soap suds into it on its
wrong side, work them well in, then dry and rub in a
solution of alum. The soap is by this means decomposed,
and its oily part distributed among the fibres of the cloth.
This recipe is taken from instructions issued for guidance
of the French soldiers and National Guards during the
siege of Paris.

WET.—Exposure to wet and cold, to all the states of the
weather, climates, and seasons, forms but part of the
soldier's existence. His health necessarily suffers from
such exposure, nor can it always be avoided; as, for
example, when he is on duty, or on service. He should
be warned, however, against remaining in his wet state, if
it can possibly be avoided. In temperate climates, rheumatism and chest affections are often thus brought on; in
hot climates, fevers and dysentery—endangering, if not
destroying life.

WINES.—If soldiers could be made to believe it, the use
of light wines would be far more pleasant, and certainly
much less injurious to them, than the spirits and beer in
which so many love to indulge. In hot countries this
would be especially the case. They may be informed that
the use of the light wines of France is nothing new in our
army; that when first placed upon a permanent footing
these wines were regularly issued to them, and that at some
of our foreign stations they continue to be so still.

WOMEN.—To quote from instructions issued to the
French soldier—" Women who roam about in the vicinity
of camps should be mistrusted. They are almost always

H

diseased. A moment of weakness may suffice to convey a justly dreaded disease, the cure of which is never certain and which not only affects its immediate subjects, but their children."

WORKSHOPS.—While it is for the advantage of men, both as regards their means and their health, that they should be employed in workshops, yet there are certain evils which need to be guarded against. The chief of these include crowding, want of ventilation, and over-heatedness of the men, thus producing an atmosphere that is as injurious in its effects as it is offensive. As a rule, the " shops" of regimental tailors and shoemakers present these defects to the greatest degree ; and, to make matters worse, bits of leather and of cloth are often thrown into the fire maintained in such places, still further increasing their offensiveness. Frequent ablutions and baths are doubly necessary for the requirements of health in the men employed under such conditions.

WORRY.—Under this head a word of caution may be given to young non-commissioned officers. Soldiers, and particularly those that have not been long enlisted, or of the nervous temperament already alluded to, may not only be driven to *commit themselves*, but have their health impaired by a system of petty worry, and what is called "nagging," on account of small matters. Soldiers, after obtaining their discharge, sometimes express how painful to them was the constant watch kept over them by non-commissioned officers,—a condition which they looked upon as little else than one of continual restraint. There may be some reason to believe that in some instances this is felt to a considerable degree.

WOUNDED IN BATTLE.—*See* FIRST DRESSINGS.—In all civilised countries a special organisation exists for attending the wounded on, and removing them from, the field, so that the necessity has ceased for men engaged in combat to quit the ranks on the plea of seeing a comrade safe to the rear. Nevertheless, occasions continually arise, not only during the fight but after it is over, where the intelligent assistance of men to their wounded comrades may be extremely beneficial; and late experience has clearly shown that it is in all cases perfectly impossible, for the regular *ambulance* establishments to succour the fallen within a moderate time, however numerous and efficient their *personnel* may be. Hence the advisableness of soldiers being taught beforehand some of the more simple methods of giving help in such an emergency. Officers have naturally great repugnance against soldiers leaving the ranks during battle to escort wounded comrades to the rear. Not only is the strength of the effective force decreased in this way, but it is notorious that few of those who thus leave the ranks rejoin while the fight rages. The proportion of wounded varies greatly, according to the circumstances of the action; so also do the kind of wounds received, and the ratio of wounded to killed. Where shells are much used the killed are relatively more numerous as compared to wounded than in fights chiefly with small arms.

Wounds by Fire-arms.—If only in the fleshy part of a limb, without fracture of a bone and without much bleeding, undo or cut off the dress from over the part, bathe in cold water, and having soaked several folds of linen or other cloth in water apply it, securing it to the wound by means of a bandage, handkerchief, or other means.

Wounds with Fracture.—The injured limb must be handled with great gentleness to avoid pain to the person as much as possible and injury to the fractured member. The dress over the wound to be cut or undone. The limb to be laid out as straight as possible, and kept in that position by two or more long pieces of wood, bundles of twigs or of grass, strips of bandage or pocket-handkerchiefs, or portions of dress used as binders around the limb, thus protected to keep it steady. In fractures of one of the legs or thighs, the shortest way to secure it is to tie it to its fellow by means of a binder, or more than one, above and below the injury. Wet cloths are to be applied to the wound itself.—*See* SWORD-CUTS.

WOUNDS WITH MUCH BLEEDING.—If the blood which rushes in streams from a wound be of a dark colour, it comes from a vein; if bright red, and it comes in jets, it is from an artery. If in either case a man could but have self-possession, the best plan is to press the point from which the blood is seen escaping with a finger or with a pellet of wet cloth, and hold either there until a surgeon comes or the wounded man can be taken to the rear. If men were taught beforehand to apply a *tourniquet* to the limb, or even to put on a handkerchief and twist it with a pinion, the plan would be to use one both above and below the seat of wound if possible to do so. It is almost needless to say that in all cases of severe bleeding the aid of the surgeon is of vital importance to the wounded man. He may and will, unless properly treated, rapidly bleed to death.—*See* HÆMORRHAGE.

LONDON : BAILLIERE, TINDALL, AND COX, KING WILLIAM STREET, STRAND.

A GUIDE TO HEALTH:

FOR THE USE OF SOLDIERS.

A

GUIDE TO HEALTH:

For the Use of Soldiers.

BY

SURGEON-MAJOR R. C. EATON,

MEDICAL STAFF.

" Life is not to live, but to be well."—MARTIAL.

CASSELL. & COMPANY, LIMITED:

LONDON, PARIS & MELBOURNE.

1890.

CONTENTS.

SECTION IV.

AIR, VENTILATION, AND SUN-LIGHT.

SECTION V.

FOOD AND CLOTHING.

SECTION VI.

DRINKS AND TOBACCO.

SECTION VII.

EXERCISE AND SLEEP.

PREFACE.

———◦◦◦———

THE object aimed at in this little work is to instruct the
soldier in preserving his health and in promoting his
physical development, whereby he may increase not only
his own well-being and comfort, but his efficiency in the
Service.

It can hardly be said that even the officers of the
Army sufficiently realise the inestimable advantages
which result from the adoption of sanitary precautions
both in barracks and camps; and among the men the
injury done by neglecting the simplest rules of health is
beyond their comprehension.

Disease cannot exist without a cause; and there is
abundant evidence that we ourselves, through ignorance
or carelessness of the laws of life and health, are
answerable for the vast majority of the ailments which
afflict us.

In compiling this little book, the following authors
have been consulted:—"Parkes' Practical Hygiene"

(De Chaumont), " Principles of Hygiene" (Willoughby), "The Book of Health" (Morris), "Hygiene and Public Health" (L. C. Parkes), "The Hygiene of Armies in the Field" (Rawlinson), "Madras Manual of Hygiene" (King), "On Disorders of Digestion" (Lauder Brunton), "Energy in Nature" (Carpenter), "Health" (Wilson), "Epidemics of the Middle Ages" (Hecker), "Edinburgh Health Lectures," "An Account of Lazarettos" (Howard), and various Health pamphlets.

A GUIDE TO HEALTH:

FOR THE USE OF SOLDIERS.

———◆◇◆———

SECTION I.

INTRODUCTORY.

THE human body is a most wonderful, complex, and perfect machine, within which its several organs are continually performing the various functions of life. Each organ fulfils its own special duty, but perfect health is only possible when they all work in harmony; because derangement of one organ is almost certain to throw the others out of gear. A vigorous and healthy life is the result of the proper and harmonious performance of all the bodily functions.

The human machine requires a sufficient supply of fuel to enable it to perform its work; and it has been found that a healthy man, under ordinary circumstances, will consume nearly a ton and a half of material in the shape of solid food, air, and water in the course of a year. Nor is this too much when we consider the enormous amount of incessant work which the functions of his body entail.

We learn from scientific calculations that the *energy* or *power of doing work* which an average man exhibits in the twenty-four hours is equal to 3,400 foot-tons—that is to say, the total force he expends in his work of twenty-four hours would raise 3,400 tons one foot from the ground. Of this amount of force about one-tenth is used in the external movements of the body, the remaining nine-tenths being required for doing the vast amount of *internal* work, such as the movements of the heart and lungs, the digestion of the food, &c., and maintaining the heat of the body at its natural standard —98·5 Fahr.

It may be interesting to observe that the work performed by a man's heart in the twenty-four hours is equal to raising 124 tons one foot high; that the force he expends daily in keeping himself warm is represented by a power sufficient to raise 2,800 tons one foot; and that the work of his chest and lungs is estimated at 21 foot-tons. So that our daily life represents an amount of work which would be almost incredible were it not that the accuracy of these calculations has been proved by the experiments of Professor Haughton and other scientific observers.

A close resemblance is said to exist between the

living machinery and that of the steam-engine. The force which moves the steam-engine is the result of the combustion of fuel by combination with the oxygen of the air drawn into the furnace ; the force which maintains the heat of the body and performs the other acts of life is derived from the combustion of food by union with the oxygen of the air taken into the body by the lungs during breathing. Here, however, the resemblance ceases, for there is no machine made by human hands which is capable of executing its own repairs, or of increasing in size and strength—growing.

Contrasting the working power of the steam-engine with that of the human body, Sir William Armstrong* says : "Observe how superior the result is in Nature's engine to what it is in ours. Nature only uses heat of a low grade, such as we find wholly unavailable. We reject our steam as useless at a temperature which would cook the animal substance, while Nature works with a heat so mild as not to hurt the most delicate tissue. And yet, notwithstanding the high-grade temperature, the quantity of work performed by the living engine, relative to the fuel consumed, puts the steam-engine to shame."

The main conditions under which the human machine is enabled to do the greatest possible amount of work,

* Now Lord Armstrong.

both mental and physical, for the longest period, are
based upon very definite principles, and can be laid
broadly down.   Briefly they are the following :—

I.

The most scrupulous cleanliness of person, clothing,
and surroundings.

II.

Abundance of pure air to breathe, by night as well
as by day.   Every occupied room ought to have direct
communication with the outside atmosphere, and ought
to be so constructed as to secure a constant supply of
fresh air without unpleasant draughts.

III.

Sunlight is as necessary as air for healthy growth
and development.   Human beings, like plants, grow
pale and sickly when deprived of it.

IV.

A sufficient quantity of wholesome and well-cooked
food is required to furnish material for the growth and
repair of the body, and the production of heat and other
forms of force.

V.

Regular and moderate exercise, with due alternation
of periods of rest, promotes a healthy and vigorous state

of body and mind. The best exercises are those which call into play all the bodily and mental functions and faculties.

VI.

Clothing is necessary to protect the body from cold and variations of temperature. The garments should be so made as to admit of the freest movements of the limbs, and to avoid injurious pressure upon any part or organ.

In order to learn the practical application of these conditions to the preservation of health, the promotion of physical and mental development, the prevention of disease, and prolongation of life, it is requisite that the reader should acquire a general but clear knowledge of the structure, mechanism, and vital functions of the human machinery.

SECTION II.

THE SKELETON—JOINTS—MUSCLES—NERVES.

THE solid framework of the body is made up of about 210 separate bones, the whole of which is familiarly called the *skeleton*. This bony frame forms a combined lever apparatus, a passive apparatus of motion.

The spinal column, or back-bone, may be considered as the foundation of the skeleton, because the different parts of the framework are connected with it as a common centre. Thus, on its upper extremity it supports the skull; laterally, it gives attachment to the ribs, through which it receives the weight of the upper limbs; inferiorly, the column is wedged in between the haunch-bones, which transmit the weight of the body to the lower limbs.

The spine, being the centre of all the movements of the body, must be pliant and flexible, yet firm to preserve the erect attitude, and to give sufficient protection to the spinal marrow, which it encloses. It is composed of 26 bones, called *vertebræ*, piled one on the other, and joined together by elastic pads of gristle; these not only connect the vertebræ together, but act as buffers to prevent shocks being transmitted through the spine to the brain.

The skull, including the face, is constructed of 22 bones. Of these, 8 go to form a beautifully firm case for the protection of the brain, while 14 enter into the formation of the face. All these bones are more or less firmly united one with the other, except the lower jaw, which is provided with most varied and complex movements for the mastication of the food.

The ribs are 24 in number, arranged 12 on each side. They form, with the vertebræ behind, and the breast-bone and rib-cartilages in front, the cavity of the chest, in which are lodged the heart and lungs.

A flat muscular partition, called the *midriff* or *diaphragm*, divides the cavity of the chest from that of the abdomen, which contains the organs of digestion. The diaphragm is the chief agent by which we inspire, or " take in a breath."

Below the abdomen is a basin-shaped cavity—the pelvis—formed laterally and in front by the two massive haunch-bones, and behind by the termination of the spinal column.

On the outside of each haunch-bone is a deep cup-like socket, which receives the rounded head of the thigh-bone, and forms the hip-joint.

The two pairs of limbs—the arms and legs—are

B

constructed on the same model, with certain modifications which are necessary for the different purposes
they are destined to subserve.   The upper limbs are
possessed of great freedom of movement in various
directions ; and thus the arm can be more efficiently
used as a protection to the head and body generally,
and the hand is enabled to fulfil its important duties of
grasping and touch.

The lower limbs being designed to sustain the weight
of the body, and convey it from place to place, it is
necessary that their bones should be of great strength ;
and this we find is the case, the bones of the thigh,
leg, and foot being remarkably strong and massive.

The bones of the foot are arranged so as to form a
very powerful arch, extending from the heel to the base
of the toes, and supporting on its summit the entire
weight of the body.   The hinder pier of the arch is
formed by two large bones, while the front pier is made
up of several smaller bones—an arrangement which gives
firmness and stability to the heel, and spring and elasticity to the front of the foot.

The *Joints* are formed between the bones, and include various degrees, as well as forms, of movement ;
in some the amount of motion is extremely limited,
while in others it is free and complete.

Joints, such as those of the elbow, knee, ankle, and

fingers, are called "hinge-joints," because they work after the manner of a door on its hinges, admitting only of a to-and-fro movement. The joints which admit of the greatest variety and extent of motion are the ball-and-socket joints, as seen in the shoulder and hip. Another form of joint—the pivot joint—is illustrated when we turn the wrist or nod the head.

The opposed surfaces of the bones entering into the formation of a joint are covered with a layer of exceedingly smooth elastic gristle, and this is lined by a delicate membrane which pours out a glairy fluid, popularly called "joint-oil." The use of this fluid is to lubricate the interior of the joint, so as to enable the opposed surfaces to work smoothly upon each other.

The ends of the bones forming the joint are kept in position by strong membranous bands, called *ligaments*, and are more or less supported by the surrounding structures.

The *Muscles* constitute the fleshy covering of the skeleton, and give to the different regions of the body their special contour and outline. They are the agents by which the active movements of the body are performed. These movements are brought about by contraction of the muscles—that is, shortening their length—so that the bones between which they are fixed are pulled upon and drawn for a time nearer together.

The majority of the muscles are attached to the bones through the intervention of *tendons* (or sinews), which occupy but a small space as they pass from the bulky muscle to the parts upon which they are designed to act, as the fingers and toes.

The muscles, together with the bones and sinews, are arranged in various mechanical contrivances, whereby efficiency of muscular action and economy of power are both secured.

There are two distinct kinds of muscles—voluntary and involuntary. The former derive their name from the fact that they are under the control of the will, and can be used when we like, such as those of the arms and legs, and of the body generally. The involuntary muscles act independently of the will, and discharge various important duties in the economy of life ; they form the muscular walls of the heart, of the blood-vessels, of the stomach, of the intestines, and of some other parts.

The voluntary muscles of the body are brought under the control of the will through the medium of the *nerves*, which communicate, like a set of telegraph wires, between the brain and the several muscles to which they are distributed.

SECTION III.

CLEANLINESS OF SKIN, HAIR, NAILS, TEETH,
CLOTHING, AND SURROUNDINGS.

THE duties of the skin in relation to health are of the greatest importance. It is not only a protective investment which covers the whole surface of the body, but it regulates the bodily heat, and acts as a purifier of the blood.

The outer layer of the skin—called the scarf-skin—is dense and hard, especially where it is exposed to friction, as in the palms of the hands and soles of the feet. Beneath it lies the true skin, which, being richly supplied with blood-vessels and nerves, is highly sensitive. Between the two skins there is a layer of cells containing colouring matter, which causes the various shades of complexion in the different races of man. The shade is deepest when the particles of colouring matter are most abundant, as is the case in the negro.

Imbedded deep down in the skin are numerous little sweat glands; these consist of coiled-up tubes, which, after a spiral course through the substance of the skin, terminate on its surface by openings called *pores*. There

are about 2,500,000 of these pores on the surface of a
man's body ; and if the glands were uncoiled and placed
one after the other, they would form a tube twenty-eight
miles in length.

Through this drainage system there is constantly
going on an exudation of watery fluid, or sweat, containing various waste-matters derived from the worn-out
tissues of the body.   The evaporation of this fluid from
the surface serves to maintain the uniform temperature
of health, and at the same time it relieves the blood of
a large quantity of impurities.

Besides the sweat glands, there are others opening
on the surface, called oil glands ; these produce an
oily substance, which aids in preserving the softness and
elasticity of the skin.

The total quantity of water and solids which thus
escapes from the surface of the body varies greatly,
according to the heat of the atmosphere, the fluids
drunk, and exercise taken ; but a healthy man, under
ordinary conditions of life, gives off from his skin daily,
in the form of sweat, about two pints of water, about
300 grains of solid matter (organic impurities), and
about 400 grains of carbonic acid.

To maintain the skin in activity and health, it must
be kept scrupulously clean.   When the body is not
regularly washed, the solid constituents of the perspira-

tion or sweat accumulate on the surface and block up the pores, thus obstructing the natural and healthy action of the sweat glands.

This arrest of the ordinary work of these glands produces skin diseases; and the blood, not being relieved of its impurities, falls gradually into an unhealthy condition, and is apt to cause fevers and other ailments.

Besides personal ill-health, the owner of a dirty skin becomes a serious nuisance, if not an actual danger, to the health of others. "The great sanitary law," said Sir Lyon Playfair, "is 'wash and be clean'; and anything which stood in the way of observance of that law impaired the health of all communities."

Water alone is not sufficient to maintain the skin in a healthy state; plenty of soap and strong rubbing must also be employed, in order that the deposit of sweat and greasy matters may be dissolved and washed off. A warm bath is more effectual in cleansing the skin than a cold one; but it is not so bracing, and is better adapted to relieve the feeling of great fatigue that follows prolonged exertion. We are told that Napoleon used to have recourse to a warm bath after the fatigue of a battle, and found it more refreshing than even sleep.

All men in health should take a cold bath or cold

sponge every morning, with a warm or tepid bath once a week as a periodical cleanser. Nothing is more invigorating to the nervous system than the " morning cold tub," and its daily use enables the body to resist the effects of sudden changes of temperature.

A useful substitute for the sponge bath consists in wringing a rough towel out of cold or tepid water, and vigorously rubbing the whole surface of the body with it.

The Turkish bath, followed by the cold douche, is admirably adapted for cleansing the skin, and is found beneficial to persons of sedentary habits, and to those whose skins do not naturally act well ; but it ·does not agree with everyone, and should only be used under medical advice.

As regards open-air bathing, the sea is more invigorating than the river or lake. The saltness of the sea water and the pure sea air tend to promote the appetite, to strengthen the muscles, and to impart a healthy tone to the nervous system.

The following simple rules, drawn up by the Royal Humane Society, should be observed by all bathers :—

1. Never bathe within two hours after a meal.

2. Never bathe when exhausted or in ill-health. The practice of plunging into water after exercise is to be thoroughly condemned.

3. Never bathe when the body is cooling after perspiration.

4. A morning bathe may be taken by those who are strong and healthy before breakfast on an empty stomach.

5. The young, or those who are delicate, should bathe two or three hours after a meal, and in the forenoon, if possible.

6. The signs which forbid open-air bathing altogether are chilliness and shivering after entering the water, numbness of hands and feet, and deficient circulation generally.

7. When the body is warm, bathing may be indulged in, provided undressing is quickly accomplished, and the body is not chilled before entering the water.

8. On leaving the water, dry and dress *quickly.* Standing about undressed, after leaving the water, is, under any circumstances, injurious.

9. Rather cut short, than prolong, the bathe. Swimmers possess the power of remaining in the water for a considerable time, in consequence of their active movements. But even in their case injury is often wrought by unduly extending the exercise. The slightest feeling of chilliness should be taken as a sign to leave the water at once.

10. Lastly: we may repeat the wholesome advice that those who experience any disagreeable symptoms after bathing—such as palpitation, giddiness, &c.—should not again enter the water without consulting a doctor.

The *Hair* is an appendage of the skin, and being a natural adornment, generally receives a fair share of attention. From a health point of view, the chief requirement is cleanliness. It should be cut short once a fortnight—a practice which not only facilitates cleanliness, but tends to strengthen the after-growth. When short, the hair may be washed with soap and water daily, but after washing it should be thoroughly dried, and a little oil or pomatum used, to supply the place of the natural oil which has been washed off.

Regarding the use of the hair-brush and comb, Dr. Jamieson, in his "Edinburgh Health Lecture," says: "Brushing should be gentle, and a brush with bristles which are neither too stiff nor too closely set should be chosen. A hard brush breaks and bruises the hair, although it seems to be doing good by scraping off a cloud of dust. One is apt to forget that the scurf re-forms faster than ever when thus roughly scratched away. Use, then, a soft brush, and use it gently. And wash the head once a week or fortnight, if not habitually daily. The teeth of the comb should not have sharp points, as these tear the skin of the head. A small tooth comb should never be used."

The *Nails*, which protect the sensitive tips of the fingers and toes, require the bestowal of some care and attention on their culture. The under surface of the free edge of the nail should never be scraped or picked with a knife, but washed with soap and water and a soft brush. The finger nails should be cut round, and the toe nails straight across. To prevent a painful affection known by the term "agnail," the skin at the roots of the nails should be gently pushed back after each time the hands are washed.

In the German army, where every little detail is attended to, the barber of each battalion is held responsible that the men's toe nails are properly cut and that their feet are kept clean and healthy.

The *Teeth* are most important agents in the work of digestion, and their preservation is therefore an important element in the preservation of health. The first step in the digestive process is the grinding of the food by the teeth, which is called mastication, and if this, either from habit or unsound teeth, be imperfectly performed, indigestion, with all its accompanying evils, is sure to follow. Slow and careful mastication is essential in order that the food may be reduced to that state in which it can be most readily and perfectly acted upon by the different digestive fluids with which it afterwards comes in contact.

When the teeth are neglected, particles of animal and vegetable food lodge between them, and undergo a process of fermentation which develops acids that injure the enamel and eventually destroy the teeth.   Against this form of decay scrupulous cleanliness is evidently the best preservative.   The mouth should be rinsed out after each meal, and the teeth should be cleaned by brushing every part of them night and morning with soap and water or a good tooth-powder, such as camphorated chalk.

Cleanliness of Clothing.—The under-clothing absorbs and retains the exudations from the skin, which tend to decompose and become offensive ; for this reason such articles as shirt, vest, drawers, and socks should be frequently changed and washed.   The under-clothing worn during the day should be removed at bed-time, to be replaced by cotton night-shirts.   This allows the day garment to get dry and aired during the hours of sleep. Dr. Parkes says : " In time of war, shirts may be partially cleaned in this way : The soldier should wear one and carry one ; every night he should change ; hang up the one he takes off to dry, and in the morning beat it out and shake it thoroughly.   In this way much dirt is got rid of.   He should then carry this shirt in his pack during the day, and substitute it for the other at night."

The outer garments also get more or less impregnated with perspiration, and require to be aired and dried from time to time, so as to get rid of all moisture.

The bed-clothes which have been in use during the night should be exposed to the air for a few hours before being re-arranged. This salutary practice not only frees them from the exhalations which they absorb from the skin and lungs, but greatly adds to the comfort of the bed at night and conduces to sound sleep.

Cleanliness of Surroundings.—Scrupulous attention to the cleansing of habitations, including the removal of slops, refuse, excreta, &c., is a matter of the utmost importance to health. The great principle is that all should be rapidly and completely removed from the house and its vicinity, " so that neither air, water, nor soil shall be made impure." The water method of removal is the cleanest and most convenient, especially where there is a good supply of water, sufficient outfall, and means of disposing of the sewage. The dry earth method is that which is usually adopted in India, and has many advantages.

Decaying animal matters being the natural food of plants, their ultimate disposal should consist in applying them to the fertilisation of land, thus converting them from dangerous impurities into wholesome food.

The diseases which have been shown to arise from

imperfect systems of sewage removal are enteric fever, dysentery, diarrhœa, cholera, yellow fever, diphtheria, sore throat, and an aggravation of other diseases.

Dust-bins ought to be especially attended to, otherwise they become sources of danger. The disposal of all kinds of refuse by burning with special apparatus is being tried in several large towns, and the plan seems likely to be a complete success.

It may be here stated that *disinfectants* are useful as adjuncts to cleanliness, but they can never be substituted for it.

The best means of purifying a foul atmosphere is by the freest possible ventilation.

SECTION IV.

AIR, VENTILATION, SUNLIGHT.

AIR is the first necessity of life. We can exist without water for days, and without food for weeks, but the air around us we must breathe, or die.

We breathe for the purpose of freeing the blood from the waste products of the body, the retention of which in the system would be prejudicial to health, if not destructive of life. During the act of breathing the blood charged with the decaying matters from the worn-out tissues is exposed to the purifying action of the air in the lungs ; by this contact with the air, the blood gives off carbonic acid, organic matters, and watery vapours, which are expelled by the windpipe, and absorbs oxygen from the freshly-inspired air.

But if the atmosphere is impure, as in rooms where there is not sufficient ventilation, the necessary purification of the blood cannot take place.

When a number of people are collected together in a badly-ventilated room, the air of that room quickly becomes impure by the accumulation of carbonic acid and organic vapours given off from the lungs and skins of the occupants. Breathing such an atmosphere for even a few hours produces headache, nausea, and other feverish symptoms; and the continued re-breathing of the same air renders it in the highest degree poisonous.

Of this we have two sad instances on record. On the night of the 18th of June, 1756, one hundred and forty-six prisoners, including one woman, were thrust into a dungeon, the Black Hole of Calcutta—a place 18 feet by 14 feet, and having but two small windows, and so densely packed, that the door had to be pressed on the last to enter.

The atmosphere of this confined place speedily became poisoned with carbonic acid and organic impurities; and the result was, that only twenty-three survived the horrors of that night. The few survivors, from what they suffered, called the place "hell in miniature."

Again, on the 1st of December, 1848, the steamer *Londonderry* was crossing the Irish Channel, when, a storm coming on, the one hundred and fifty passengers were confined below the hatches, which were battened down. Of these persons, seventy were poisoned by the impure air.

Living habitually in an atmosphere more moderately tainted with the products of respiration tends to produce consumption and other lung diseases. The late Sir

James Clark has said: " If an infant, born in perfect
health and of the healthiest parents, be kept in close
rooms, in which ventilation and cleanliness are neglected,
a few months will often suffice to produce consumptive
disease." Dr. Parkes, too, states : " The average mortality
in this country increases tolerably regularly with density
of population. Density of population usually implies
poverty, and insufficient food, and unhealthy work, but
its main concomitant condition is impurity of air from
overcrowding, deficiency of cleanliness, and imperfect
removal of excreta ; and when this condition is removed
a very dense and poor population may be perfectly
healthy."

Further, overcrowded and ill-ventilated places tend
to increase the virulence and spread of infectious
diseases.

From these simple facts we learn the importance of
having pure air to breathe, and, therefore, of the free
ventilation of our dwellings.

Doors, windows, and chimneys should be utilised as
aids in the work of ventilation. In summer, the passage
of a natural stream of fresh air through open doors and
windows is the most efficient means of ventilating a
room ; in winter, the chimney in a room in which a fire
is burning forms an excellent ventilator.

The essential points are to provide outlets for the

C

escape of foul air, and inlets for the admission of fresh air.

The foul air, heated by lights and by being breathed ascends; therefore the outlets should be near the ceiling. The inlets should be 9 or 10 feet from the floor, unless when the air is warmed before admission; then the inlets may be at the bottom of the room.

Every window in the house should be kept open an inch or two at the top, or, as suggested by Dr. Hinckes Bird—" Raise the lower sash a few inches, and fill up the vacant space with a block of wood, so that the lower sash will rest upon it. The result will be that a current of air flows in between the bottom of the upper sash and the top of the lower sash without draught or annoyance."

Bedrooms require to be supplied with fresh air not only during the day, but whilst we are asleep. At night the windows should be kept slightly open at the top in winter, and wide open in summer. In addition, every room should be flushed through with air, when not occupied, by opening freely the doors and windows. By this means the organic matters and other impurities floating in the atmosphere of the apartment are carried off, and their poisonous qualities completely destroyed.

The sense of smell gives a fair idea of the amount of impurities in the air of a dwelling-room, but it is necessary that the observer should enter the room after being some time in the open air, because breathing foul air rapidly destroys the perception of its foulness.

It is estimated that the quantity of pure air that should pass through an inhabited room in order to maintain the atmosphere in a condition fit for breathing is 3,000 cubic feet per head per hour.

In this climate, it has been found by experiment that the air of a room cannot be changed more frequently than three times per hour without causing an unpleasant draught; therefore, each person ought to have a breathing space of 1,000 cubic feet. That is, a room 10 feet square by 10 feet high represents the amount of superficial area and cubic space which should be allotted to each individual, and the air of this room should be changed three times per hour.

Howard, the great philanthropist and reformer of prisons, so long ago as a century, said: "It may be asked of what size I would wish prisoners' solitary *night rooms* to be ? I answer, ten feet long, ten feet high, and eight feet wide." At the present day the cubic space allotted to each man in barracks is only 600 cubic feet.

In estimating the quantity of air to be supplied to inhabited rooms, fires and lights must be taken into account. A pound of coal requires 240 cubic feet of air for complete combustion, the resulting gases and other products escaping by the chimney. A common gas-burner consumes as much air as three or four men, and an ordinary oil-lamp or candle as much as two men.

The sick require a much larger supply of fresh air than healthy persons; in fact, in many diseases almost complete exposure to the air not only favours the recovery of the patients, but prevents the spread of disease.

SUNLIGHT.

Dwelling-rooms ought to be so arranged that they may receive plenty of sunlight, which, as a means of promoting a vigorous state of health, is as necessary as fresh air. This is now so fully recognised by medical men, that sun-baths are provided for the patients in many of the hospitals, both in this country and in America.

Recent experiments, conducted by Professor Tyndall, have shown that direct sunshine arrests decomposition, and has a valuable chemical power of destroying disease germs.

The Italian proverb, " Where the sun does not come the doctor does," is perfectly true.

SECTION V.

FOOD AND COOKERY.

EVERY act of life, however simple, involves destruction of tissue, wear and tear, which must be replaced by new material. In order to provide this new material to supply the place of the destroyed structures, we take food.

The purposes of food are two-fold. It supplies building material for the growth and repair of the bodily frame, and furnishes fuel for the production of heat and energy for working the human machine.

For the due performance of these purposes, four great classes of nourishment are necessary :—

1st. Nitrogenous, such as albumen, myosin, gelatin, casein, and gluten. Of these, albumen, myosin, and gelatin are derived from butcher's meat, poultry, eggs, and fish. Casein is found in milk, and gluten in most vegetable foods, notably in wheat. The special functions of the elements of this class are to build up and repair the constant waste of the body.

2nd, Fats, such as butter, lard, suet, dripping, and

vegetable oils.   These substances are the principal
sources of bodily heat and motive power.   Fat also
enters largely into the composition of all nervous structures, and it aids in the digestion of other substances
of a diet.

3rd. **Starchy** and **saccharine** : the former includes
arrowroot, sago, tapioca, corn-flour, gum, and nearly
all the farinaceous foods ; the latter consists of the
different kinds of sugar—cane, grape, beet, &c.   All
these are important articles of a diet, and greatly assist
in the production of heat and force for work.

4th. Salts and water—the former being common
salt, lime, soda, potash, magnesia, phosphates, iron, &c.
Common salt is required to promote digestion, while
the others are essential constituents of the different
structures and fluids of the body.   Water is even more
essential to life and health than food of any other class,
for without it all the others would be useless.   It enters
into every tissue, forming more than two-thirds of the
entire weight of the body ; and it is necessary for the
performance of every act of life.

A considerable amount of the water which the body
requires is supplied in the so-called " solid food."

The following Table, giving the nutritive value of
different kinds of solid food, shows that they all contain
a large percentage of water.

TABLE FOR CALCULATING DIETS.

(From "Parkes' Hygiene.")

Articles.	In 100 Parts.				
	Water.	Albuminates.	Fats.	Carbohydrates.	Salts.
Meat of best quality, with little fat, like beefsteaks, . }	74·4	20·5	3·5	...	
Uncooked meat of the kind supplied to soldiers—beef and mutton. Bone constitutes ⅕th of the soldier's allowance,[1] }	75	15	8·4	...	1.9
Uncooked meat of fattened cattle. Calculated from Lawes' and Gilbert's experiments. These numbers are to be used if the meat is very fat, ... }	63	14	19	...	3·7
Cooked meat,[2] roast, no dripping being lost. Boiled assumed to be the same, . }	54	27·6	15·45	...	2·95
Corned beef (Chicago),[3] . .	40	40	15	...	5
Salt beef (Girardin), . .	49·1	29·6	0·2	...	21·1
„ pork (Girardin), . .	44·1	26·1	7·0	...	22·8
Fat pork (Letheby), . .	39·0	9·8	48·9	...	2·3
Dried bacon (Letheby), . .	15·0	8·8	73·3	...	2·9
Smoked ham (J. König), . .	27·8	24·0	36·5	...	10·1
Horse flesh do. . .	74·3	21·7	2·6	...	1·0
White fish (Letheby), . .	78·0	18·1	2·9	...	1·2
Poultry (Letheby), . . .	74·0	21·0	3·8	...	1·0
Bread, white wheaten, of average quality, ... }	40	8	1·5	49·2	1·3
Wheat flour, average quality, .	15	11	2	70·3	1·7

[1] The gelatine of the meat is reckoned with the albuminates; it is not certain what deduction should be made on account of its lower nutritive value, which is about ⅕th that o albumen (Bischof).

[2] These numbers are taken from John Ranke's analysis.

[3] This is excellent meat, palatable and nutritious; half a pound would form an ample ration for the field, with the due proportion of biscuit, &c. As it is merely *corned* and not *salted* like ordinary salt meat, it is probable that its constituents may be allowed nearly their full nutritive value.

Articles.	In 100 Parts.				
	Water.	Albuminates.	Fats.	Carbohydrates.	Salts.
Biscuit, ...	8	15·6	1·3	73·4	1·7
Rice, ...	10	5	·8	83·2	0·5
Oatmeal (Letheby), . . .	15	12·6	5·6	63·0	3
Maize (Poggiale) (cellulose excluded), ...	13·5	10	6·7	64·5	1·4
Macaroni (König), . . .	13·1	9·0	0·3	76·8	0·8
Millet (König) (cellulose excluded),	12·3	11·3	3·6	67·3	2·3
Arrowroot, ...	15·4	0·8	...	83·3	·27
Peas (dry), ...	15	22	2	53	2·4
Potatoes, ...	74	2·0	·16	21·0	1
Carrots (cellulose excluded), .	85	1·6	·25	8·4	1·0
Cabbage, ...	91	1·8	·5	5·8	·7
Butter, ...	6	·3	91	...	variable taken as ·7
Egg (10 per cent. must be deducted for shell from the weight of the egg), . .	73·5	13·5	11·6	...	1
Cheese, ...	36·8	33·5	24·3	...	5·4
Milk (sp. gr. 1029 and over), .	86·8	4	3·7	4·8	·7
Cream (Letheby), . . .	66	2·7	26·7	2·8	1·8
Skimmed milk (Letheby), .	88	4·0	1·8	5·4	0·8
Sugar, ...	3	...	...	96·5	·5
Pemmican (de Chaumont),[1] .	7·2	35·4	55·2	...	1·8

The principles composing the four classes of nourishment must be present in certain proportions in every diet which is to maintain life in its most perfect state for a lengthened period. Excess or deficiency of any one class exercises a very unfavourable influence on health.

Although man almost universally derives his food from both the animal and vegetable kingdoms, it is quite

[1] The sweet pemmican used in the Arctic Expedition of 1875—6 was similar to the above (the ordinary pemmican used in the same expedition), with the addition of about 5 per cent. of cane sugar. In other cases, particularly in the American pemmican, raisins and currants are added. (See *Report of Committee on Scurvy* for analyses by Professor Franklin and Dr. de Chaumont.) A little pepper is added, not reckoned quantitatively in the above analysis, but probably included in the "loss," *i.e.*, the difference between the sum of the above constituents and 100.

possible for him to obtain the principles necessary for his growth and development from the vegetable world alone; but, apart from his general inclination, the construction of his digestive apparatus shows that he is designed to live on a mixture of animal and vegetable food. Moreover, a mixed diet is that which is best adapted to supply the requisite materials in proper proportion for the wants of the human body.

Milk, which is provided by Nature as the only nourishment for the young of man and beast for many months after birth, contains all the elements needed for the support of life and growth, and may be regarded as the type of what a food should be. It is not fitted, however, to be the sole food of the adult; but when taken with other articles of food—such as oatmeal porridge, bread, or rice—it is invaluable. Cow's milk is that which is most generally used for human food, but the milk of the buffalo, goat, sheep, ass, and mare, are much used in some countries, especially in India and Tartary.

Milk has the evil reputation of occasionally conveying the poisons of fevers, but this is probably always due either to adulteration with dirty water, or to "washing the cans" with that noxious element, or to the milk being exposed to an atmosphere loaded with disease germs. As a protection against the spread of fevers through the medium of milk, it should be boiled.

Exposure to the temperature of boiling water for five or ten minutes removes the injurious qualities of the milk.

The following are the physical characters of good milk, as given by Dr. Parkes :—" Placed in a narrow glass, the milk should be quite opaque, of full white colour, without deposit, without peculiar smell or taste. When boiled, it should not change in appearance."

Preserved milks are now very extensively consumed, and are most valuable when fresh milk cannot be procured.

Butter, which is the fatty portion of the milk, is the most largely used of all the animal fats. It is obtained by the process of churning, and preserved by the addition of salt, in proportion varying from two to eight per cent. Butter is wholesome and easily digested, except when it is becoming rancid. It is then liable to cause indigestion.

Margarine is manufactured from beef or mutton suet by a refining process. When made from the fresh fat of healthy animals, it forms a cheap and wholesome substitute for butter.

Cheese consists principally of the casein of milk, separated from it by the action of an acid—rennet. It contains a large amount of nutritive material in small bulk, and is a valuable article of food. The richness of the milk determines the quality of the cheese. Double

Glo'ster and Stilton are made from new milk to which cream has been added; single Glo'ster, Dutch, &c., from new milk alone; and the poorest kinds of American cheeses from *skim-milk*, or milk from which the cream has been removed.

Eggs, like milk, comprise all the materials requisite for the growth and development of the body. Newly laid eggs are the most easily digested.

A good egg is slightly transparent, and sinks in a ten per cent. solution of common salt. A doubtful egg will float in the above solution, and a bad one even in fresh water.

Our supplies of *Meat* are derived entirely from the vegetable feeders, and chiefly from the ox, sheep, and pig. There is little difference in the relative nutritive values of the flesh of these three animals; they differ only in the proportion of fat and by different degrees of digestibility. Venison and the flesh of other wild animals—game—is no less nutritious than beef or mutton, and in general it is more easily digested. Horse-flesh is extensively used on the Continent and in parts of South America, and has the reputation of being very sustaining.

The advantages of meat as an article of diet are: its composition is identical with that of the body which it is intended to nourish, it is easily cooked, and easily

digested. Its great disadvantage is the absence of
carbo-hydrates—starches and sugars; these are, therefore, supplied in a mixed diet by the addition of
potatoes, bread, or rice.

Animals intended for human food should be in sound
health, in good condition, and neither too young nor
too old. Meat should be inspected twelve or fourteen
hours after being slaughtered. The following outward
characteristics of good meat are given by Dr. Letheby,
in his " Lectures on Food ":—

" (1) It is neither of a pale pink colour nor of a
deep purple tint, for the former is a sign of disease,
and the latter indicates that the animal has not been
slaughtered, but has died with the blood in it, or has
suffered from acute fever.

" (2) It has a marbled appearance, from the ramifi-
cations of little veins of fat among the muscles.

" (3) It should be firm and elastic to the touch, and
should scarcely moisten the fingers; bad meat being
wet, and sodden, and flabby, with the fat looking like
jelly or wet parchment.

" (4) It should have little or no odour, and the odour
should not be disagreeable, for diseased meat has a
sickly, cadaverous smell, and sometimes a smell of
physic. This is very discoverable when the meat is
chopped up and drenched with warm water,

"(5) It should not shrink or waste much in cooking.

"(6) It should not run to water, or become very wet, on standing for a day or so; but should, on the contrary, be dry upon the surface.

"(7) When dried at a temperature of 212°, or thereabouts, it should not lose more than seventy to seventy-four per cent. of its weight, whereas bad meat will often lose as much as 80 per cent."

Poultry—fowls, turkeys, etc.—and rabbits are equally nutritious with butcher's meat, but they are deficient both in fats and salts. Hence it is usual to combine bacon, ham, or tongue with them to supply the deficiency. The flesh of ducks and geese is very rich in fats, and consequently liable to disagree with delicate stomachs.

Fish, as a general rule, is one of the most wholesome, nutritious, and easily digested of foods. It is valuable not only as an addition to other foods, but as a substitute for meat. The composition of white fish approaches most nearly to lean beef, as shown in the following tables of analyses by Dr. Pavy:—

	Lean Beef.	Fat Beef.	White Fish.
Nitrogenous or flesh-forming matter	19·3	14·8	18·1
Fat	3·6	29·8	2·9
Minerals	5·1	4·4	1·0
Water	72·0	51·0	78·0
	100·0	100·0	100·0

White fish, such as sole, turbot, whiting, plaice, &c., are more easily digested than the rich and oily fishes—salmon, eels, mackerel, herrings, &c. These latter contain from five to fourteen per cent. of fat, and are superior in nutritive power to the white varieties.

Shell-fish contain much valuable nutriment, but they are often found to disagree, and should therefore be used with caution. Oysters in the raw state are the most wholesome and digestible of the ordinary kinds of shell-fish.

The *Crustaceans*, as the lobster, crab, cray-fish, shrimp, and prawn, are highly nutritious, but rather indigestible.

It is most essential that every description of fish intended for human food should be perfectly fresh and " in season."

VEGETABLE FOOD.

There are two classes of vegetable foods—cereals and legumes. Of the cereals, wheat, oats, barley, rye, Indian corn, and rice are the most important. From wheat is prepared the flour of which *bread*, the principal food of mankind, is made. When the wheat grain is ground and sifted, it is separated into two substances—the outer covering, called *bran*, and the inner portion, called *flour*. The bran, though not devoid of nutriment, is to a great extent indigestible, and is used chiefly as food for cattle.

The flour is reduced to varying degrees of fineness, known as superfine, seconds or middlings, pollards or thirds, or bran flour. The fine and white kinds of flour are more palatable and more nutritious than the coarse varieties.

Good flour should be quite white ; any decided yellow tinge shows commencing changes and unfitness for use. It should be free from grittiness, sour taste, or mouldy smell.

In making bread, the usual proportions in England are—flour, 20 lbs. ; tepid water, 8 to 12 lbs. (6½ to 9½ pints) ; yeast, 4 ounces ; to which a little mashed potato is added, and 1½ to 2 ounces of salt. One sack (280 lbs.) will make from 90 to 105 loaves ; or 100 lbs. of flour will make 129 to 150 lbs. of bread.

In order to obtain good bread, the ingredients must be sound and genuine ; they must be skilfully inter-mixed, the dough thoroughly kneaded, and the process of baking conducted at an uniform temperature of 212° Fahr. The crust of the baked loaf should amount to 30 per cent. of the weight ; it should be crisp and well-browned, but not charred. The small cellular cavities in the crumb should be regular and present in every part ; the walls of these cavities should not be tough. The colour should be white or brownish, in proportion to the admixture of bran. There should be no sour taste even if the bread is held in the mouth for a considerable time.

Heavy and sodden bread is very indigestible, and indicates bad flour, bad yeast, or faulty preparation.

Bread is more digestible when toasted, but the toast should be eaten soon after it is made, otherwise it becomes tough and leathery.

Being deficient in fat, bread requires the addition of butter, fat bacon, or margarine to make it a complete food.

Plain biscuits are simply flour and water mixed, and baked at a high temperature. From being well dried and baked, they are, bulk for bulk, more nutritious than bread, in the proportion of 3 to 4. They are very portable, and possess the great advantage of keeping ; but as a staple article of food they are incapable of replacing bread, except temporarily.

Sweet Biscuits are made by the addition of milk, butter, eggs, sugar, &c.

The Indian Chupatty, which forms the principal food of large populations in the North-west, consists merely of wheat flour, water, and salt. It requires to be slowly baked, at a temperature not exceeding that of boiling water. With the addition of butter or *ghee*, it is palatable and nutritious.

Macaroni and *Vermicelli* are made from wheat flour

rich in gluten. They contain a large amount of nutriment in small bulk, and are capable of being cooked in a variety of ways.

Oatmeal is highly nutritious, and has the advantage of being economical. Dr. Parkes kept a strong soldier doing hard work in perfect health on $1\frac{3}{4}$ lbs. of oatmeal and 2 pints of milk daily, at a cost of fivepence for the meal and fourpence for the milk. The man himself was sorry to return to his soldier's ration of bread and meat.

"Oatmeal is especially the food of the people of Scotland, and was formerly that of the northern parts of England—counties which have always produced as healthy and as vigorous a race of men as any other in Europe." (Cullen.) It cannot be made into bread, like wheat flour, but is used in the form of porridge or cakes. Made into a drink with water and sugar, oatmeal is found to possess great sustaining powers in hard work. The proportions are $\frac{1}{4}$ lb. of oatmeal to 3 quarts of water; it should be well boiled, and then $1\frac{1}{2}$ oz. of brown sugar added. Before drinking shake up the oatmeal well through the liquid. In summer, drink it cold; in winter, hot. (Parkes.)

Barley is now rarely used in England as an article of food, but is largely employed for brewing and distilling purposes. It is rich in phosphoric acid and iron, and very nutritious. The grain, deprived of its

D

husk and rounded, is called " Pearl Barley," and is much used as an addition to soups, and for making drinks for invalids.

Rye makes a sour, heavy bread, well known in Germany as " Schwartzbrod," or black bread. It is apt to disagree with those unaccustomed to its use.

Indian Corn, or *Maize*, ranks high in nutritive value, and contains six or seven per cent. of fat. It is extensively used as an article of food both in this country and America. The meal is generally eaten in the form of porridge, and requires very careful cooking to render it digestible. It should be steeped in water for two or three hours, and then boiled for two or three hours at a moderate heat. The young green ears (cobs) make a delicious vegetable when boiled in milk or water. Maize flour, deprived of its harsh flavour by a chemical process, forms the articles sold under the names of " Corn-flour," " Oswego," " Maizena," &c., so much used in the preparation of puddings. " Polenta," which is a favourite dish with the Italian peasantry, is a porridge made with Indian meal and cheese or chestnuts. The " Jonny Cakes " of America are composed chiefly of Indian meal.

Rice is the staple food of the natives of India and China, but in Europe is used more as a luxury than a food. Marsden, in his " History of Sumatra," says:

" Rice is the grand material of food on which a hundred millions of the inhabitants of the earth subsist, and although chiefly confined by nature to the regions included between and bordering on the tropics, its cultivation is probably more extensive than that of wheat, which the Europeans are wont to consider as the universal staff of life." In composition, it is poor in nitrogenous substances, but rich in starch, and has the advantage of being easily digested. Rice-flour may be made into cakes, but does not admit of being made into bread, unless when mixed with wheat-flour and other things. Rice should be thoroughly cooked by boiling or steaming, the latter being the preferable method.

There are several other varieties of grain used in India and Africa, but in this country they are almost unknown.

The Legumes include peas, beans, lentils, &c. Of these, peas are the most extensively consumed, and may be regarded as a type of the class ; they contain a large amount of nutritious matter, and when young and green are easily digested. The meal of the dried pea, if thoroughly boiled, forms a nutritive addition to soup. A valuable concentrated food—Erbswurst—is made by mixing together, cooking, and baking pea-flour, meat, and fat, with a little salt and pepper. It can readily be made into a palatable and nutritious soup. The exact process of manufacturing Erbswurst is not published.

Potatoes constitute a wholesome and popular article of food ; they contain a large proportion of starch and some valuable anti-scorbutic salts. Their absolute nutritive value is not great, but when eaten with fat bacon or butter, they are capable of sustaining life and vigour. Potatoes should be boiled in their skins ; otherwise their flavour is injured, and a large proportion of the salts passes into the water. Steaming is the most economical method of cooking them.

Cabbages, carrots, parsnips, turnips, and other succulent vegetables, contain very little nutriment, but are valuable chiefly on account of their anti-scorbutic properties ; they are also useful for imparting flavour and variety to other articles of greater nutritive value. Stale vegetables are to be avoided, as they undergo changes similar to those which take place in animal food, and are liable to produce derangement of the digestive organs. As regards compressed vegetables, it is extremely doubtful whether they possess any anti-scorbutic properties whatever. When fresh vegetables are not procurable, lime-juice should be substituted.

Condiments, such as mustard, pepper, vinegar sauces, &c., whilst having no nutritive value of their own, add flavour to insipid substances, and stimulate appetite and digestion. They should, however, be used in moderation, for when taken in excess they act injuriously on the digestive organs.

AMOUNT OF FOOD REQUIRED.

The *quantity* and *kind of food* required to sustain life in a healthy condition must necessarily vary according to age, exercise, and climate.

In early life, growth and development must be provided for in addition to the other requirements of the body. A growing lad, as a recruit, whose frame is being gradually developed in size and stature, ought to have a daily allowance of from 60 to 70 ounces of solid food, of which about one-fourth should be meat.

At maturity there is less demand for the materials of growth, and, therefore, the relative proportion of animal food should be considerably reduced.

For an average man, doing a moderate amount of work in a temperate climate, the following may be accepted as a fair example of a simple form of mixed diet :—Meat (uncooked), 1lb. ; Bread, 1½lbs. ; Butter, 1½ ounces ; Potatoes, 12 ounces ; Milk, 9 ounces ; Sugar, 1 ounce ; Salt, ½ ounce. In addition to this, from 40 to 80 ounces of Water are required in some form or other. In a state of absolute rest a much smaller supply of food will suffice. On the other hand, very hard labour demands an increase of food in proportion to the work done.

The careful experiments of two German chemists have shown that the internal and external work of the body is done chiefly at the expense of the fats, starches, gums, &c., and that during great physical exertion not so much extra meat as vegetable food is required.

Climate influences the demand for food, and Nature implants in man a desire for that kind of food which is most in harmony with the wants of his system. Fats and oils are the most powerful heat-producers, and are, therefore, largely consumed by the inhabitants of cold climates. Dr. Kane, in his "Arctic Explorations," says:— "Our journeys have taught us the wisdom of the Eskimo appetite, and there are few among us who do not relish a slice of raw blubber or a chunk of frozen walrus beef. The liver of a walrus (aracktanak), eaten with little slices of his fat, of a verity is a delicious morsel."

In the tropics meat is sparingly used, vegetable food —such as rice in India—forming the chief article of native diet. The splendid races of Northern India live almost entirely on whole-meal cakes, with a little butter or ghee, and can walk fifty or sixty miles a day on this diet.

But in no circumstances should natural appetite be disregarded, for, as Dr. Lauder Brunton remarks :—" In a healthy man, the best guide, both as to quantity and quality, is appetite. Food that is eaten with a relish is, as a rule, wholesome ; and sometimes it is rather astonishing to find how people's instincts guide them to what is suitable for them, in utter defiance of all *à priori* notions."

Or, as Dr. Arthur Flint puts it:—" The diet should be regulated by the appetite, the palate, and by common sense." The old rule laid down by Hippocrates "that there must be an exact balance between food and exercise, and that disease results from excess either way," is based upon sound principles.

FREQUENCY OF MEALS.

As regards the frequency of meals, it may be stated generally that three substantial meals in the day are sufficient for adults, and that the interval between one meal and another should not exceed five or six hours. During rest and sleep there is little or no demand for food, because the functions of the body are less active, and there is less waste going on.

The usual custom—breakfast at 8 a.m., dinner at 1 p.m., and supper at 6 p.m.—is that which seems best adapted to the needs of the soldier.

ELEMENTS OF COOKERY.

Cooking consists in the application of heat in such a manner as to convert our food from its raw state to a condition more favourable for digestion and nutrition, at the same time rendering it more acceptable to the sight and taste.

There is nothing of greater importance, as affecting the health and welfare of the soldier, than a good knowledge of the art of cookery. Badly-cooked food gives rise to indigestion, and excites a craving for strong drink ; besides, much valuable nutriment is wasted through unskilful cooking. Food that is well cooked and savoury will be appetising and digestible ; whereas the same food badly cooked and insipid will only excite disgust. Moreover, the skilful cook not only makes food tender and palatable, but provides that variety in meals which is so essential to the perfect nutrition of the body.

Dr. Lauder Brunton, in his work " On Disorders of Digestion," says :—" Some may think that, in speaking of cookery as a moral agent, I am greatly exaggerating its power ; and they may regard it as idle folly if I go still further, and say that cookery is not only a powerful moral agent in regard to individuals, but may be of great service in regenerating a nation. Yet, in saying this, I believe I am speaking quite within bounds, and I believe that schools of cookery for the wives of working men in this country will do more to abolish drinking habits than any number of teetotal associations."

The principal operations of cookery are boiling, roasting, baking, frying, broiling, and stewing.

Boiling.—Fresh meat should be plunged at once into boiling water, so as to form a coating of hardened albumen on the surface, which prevents the escape of the nutritive juices from the interior. After continuing the boiling for five or six minutes, the water should then be kept at a temperature not exceeding 160° Fahr., till the meat is sufficiently cooked. If the heat be excessive, the meat is rendered hard, shrunken, and tasteless.

Boiling is the most economical of the cooking processes, and boiled meats, though less savoury, are more easily digested. It is unsuited, however, to the flesh of young animals, which abounds in substances readily dissolved in water.

Salt beef, salt pork, and salt fish should be put on in cold water, and slowly boiled; the addition of a little vinegar to the water is recommended, with the view to soften the hardened texture of the meat. Fresh fish should be put on in boiling water, to which salt has been added; by this means it becomes firmer, and retains more of its flavour.

Roasting is conducted on the same principles as

boiling. To retain the soluble juices, the meat must first be subjected to a strong heat before a good open fire, and afterwards allowed to roast slowly. It is the most suitable mode of cooking ducks, geese, venison game, pork, and the flesh of young animals. The fat and other matters which exude from the meat into the dripping-pan should be used for frequent *basting*. The usual time allowed for roasting is a quarter of an hour for every pound of beef, mutton, goose, and turkey, and from seventeen to twenty minutes for every pound of pork or veal.

Baking is virtually the same as roasting, only it is done in a closed oven, and the heat is more equally maintained. The oven must be kept scrupulously clean ; otherwise the meat is liable to acquire the unpleasant flavour of burnt fat.

Frying is conducted through the medium of butter, lard, dripping, or oil, at a temperature of 380° or 400° Fahr. The frying-pan should be six inches deep, and charged with sufficient oil or fat to cover the article to be fried. The fish or meat should be immersed in the melted fat or oil at the above temperature, and left until its surface becomes a light golden brown. Good frying fat can be used repeatedly, but requires to be clarified from time to time.

Broiling is done on a grid-iron over a clear brisk fire.

The grid-iron must be heated, and the bars rubbed with a little fat before the meat or fish is put on it. A chop or steak takes from ten to twelve minutes to cook, and should be turned every two or three minutes. Steak-tongs, or a fork stuck lightly in the fat, should be used for turning, so that no gravy may escape.

Stewing is the best way of obtaining a wholesome and savoury dish at a minimum of cost. The meat is generally cut up and mixed with a large quantity of vegetables; little or no water is required—the juice of the meat and other articles being sufficient. The meat and vegetables should be placed in a saucepan in alternate layers, and allowed to stew slowly at a low heat for two hours. As a rule, tinned meats are more palatable when made into stews.

Bones contain a certain amount of nutriment, and as they form about twenty per cent. of the meat, it is desirable that they should be utilised as far as possible. They require to be broken up into small fragments, put into cold water, and slowly boiled for four or five hours. The soup resulting consists principally of gelatin dissolved in water, which alone is a very imperfect nutrient; but with the addition of groats, pearl-barley, pea-flour, or oatmeal, it can be made highly nutritious. All available scraps and trimmings of meat should be put into the pot with the bones.

SECTION VI.

DRINKS AND TOBACCO.

WATER, which is the drink provided for us by Nature, is derived from rain, springs, wells, rivers, and the distillation of sea water.

Rain water is pure and wholesome, but special care must be taken in its collection. It is liable to receive impurities from the surfaces upon which it falls, and if collected in towns or near large manufactories, it becomes tainted with the various matters contained in the smoke.

Springs are fed from subterranean reservoirs, which are themselves dependent upon the rain which percolates through the ground overlying them. The water yielded by springs is charged with gaseous and mineral matters, derived from the strata through or over which it has passed—the majority, if not the whole, of which are harmless. The deeper the source whence the water is obtained, the less liable it is to pollution from organic impurities. Springs rising from granitic, meta-morphic, or trap rock generally yield very pure and wholesome water.

Wells are artificial springs, and should be sunk as deep as possible, so as to pass through an impermeable stratum, such as sand, gravel, chalk, or granite. Water thus obtained is generally hard, but of great organic purity. The ground in the vicinity of a well ought to be kept free from animal or vegetable refuse, and the mouth of the well carefully covered and protected from external sources of impurity. Shallow wells, receiving their supply from superficial drainage, should only be used when other sources are not available. Wells in the neighbourhood of cesspools, graveyards, sewers, or badly constructed surface drains, should not be used, as they invariably contain decomposing organic matter.

River water is always more or less contaminated, especially in highly cultivated and thickly populated districts. " Nor is this to be wondered at, considering that rivers are the natural drains of the country, into which every particle of rain falling within their watersheds (except that evaporated from the surface) ultimately finds its way, with everything which it is capable of dissolving or suspending." On the other hand, the impurities are largely diluted, and river water undergoes considerable purification by natural processes. For example, the Thames water is as pure at Hampton Court as it is one hundred miles higher up, although it has received large quantities of sewage between those points.

When the supply is obtained from a running stream,

a convenient spot should be selected for taking water for drinking and cooking, another lower down for watering cattle, and a third still lower for personal ablution and washing clothes. Precautions should be taken to prevent the stream being fouled at any points above where the drinking water is procured.

Distillation is now largely used at sea and in towns on the coast where the rainfall is scanty, but the water thus obtained is insipid, owing to deficient aëration.   If, however, it is filtered through charcoal or exposed to the air in finely divided currents, it assumes the refreshing taste of spring water.

The chemical examination of water requires skill and practical knowledge, and it is extremely difficult for a person without special training to determine whether a water is good or bad.   At the same time, the physical characters of good drinking water are important, and may be a help.   Dr. Parkes lays down :—" If a water be colourless, clear, free from suspended matter, of a brilliant (or adamantine) lustre, devoid of smell or taste, except such as is recognised to be the characteristic of good potable water, we shall in the majority of cases be justified in pronouncing it a good and wholesome water ; whilst, according as it deviates from these characters, we shall be proportionately justified in regarding it with suspicion."

Water of a suspicious nature ought to be distilled, boiled, or filtered ; the two former are the most effectual, but the last has the advantage of convenience. Boiling kills most low forms of life, and is therefore a good safe-guard against the communication of disease through the medium of drinking water. Filtering through animal charcoal or spongy iron removes living organisms and suspended impurities. All filters require to be cleansed and to have the charcoal or other filtering material renewed periodically.

It is most essential to health that water should not only be good in quality, but sufficient in quantity. It is used for drinking cooking, and ablution of persons, clothes, and dwellings ; for the flushing of closets and drains ; for the drinking and washing of animals, &c.

The quantity of water required per head daily is as follows :—

Domestic use, without baths or closets . .	12 gallons.
Water-closets	6 ,,
Bathing	4 ,,
Unavoidable waste	3 ,,
	25 ,,

There are two classes of beverages which are in use in nearly every country in the world. The first includes tea, coffee, and cocoa ; the second spirits, wine, and beer.

Tea is soothing to the nervous system : it increases the action of the heart, lungs, and skin, and enables the body to resist the depressing effects of exposure and fatigue. Dr. Parkes says " that it should form the drink *par excellence* of the soldier on service. It has been found equally serviceable in the Arctic regions and in the Tropics. In the expedition to the North Pole, under Sir George Nares, tea was preferred to spirits. Captain Burnaby, in his " Ride to Kkiva," speaking of tea, says :—" This beverage becomes an absolute necessity when riding across the Steppes in mid-winter, and is far superior in heat-giving properties to any wine or spirits. In fact, a traveller would succumb to cold on the latter when the former will save his life."

Coffee, like tea, has a restorative and invigorating effect, but is more stimulating to the nervous system. It is an important article of diet for soldiers, and is said to be protective against *Malaria*. Hot coffee with bread or biscuit is invaluable for men going on early morning or night duties. Dr. Hooker states that in the Antarctic Expedition the men all preferred coffee to spirits.

It should, however, be borne in mind that the intemperate use of either tea or coffee is apt to produce sleeplessness, tremor of the muscles, and indigestion.

Cocoa differs from tea and coffee in being much more

nutritious, and is therefore useful for men undergoing great physical exertion.

Spirits, wine, and beer owe their chief effects upon the system generally, and upon the different organs of the body, to a substance contained in them called *alcohol*, which is the stimulant in all intoxicating drinks. In small quantities, and in a diluted form, alcohol taken with a meal stimulates the stomach, increasing the flow of gastric juice and aiding digestion. But where the digestion is sound and healthy, this stimulating action tends to produce injurious rather than beneficial results.

That alcohol is not a necessity in health is clearly expressed by Dr. Lauder Brunton when he says :—" So long as a man is young and healthy, he does not require alcohol, and is better without it. I think it better in every way for people to abstain entirely from the use of alcohol until they reach the age of manhood."

The experience of former campaigns goes to prove that men are more healthy, more vigorous, and better able to bear fatigues, both in hot and cold climates, without either spirits, wine, or beer. The following instances, taken from Parkes' " Practical Hygiene," may be quoted.

" In the American War of Independence in 1783, Lord Cornwallis made a march over 2,000 miles in Virginia, under the most trying circumstances of

E

exposure to cold and wet; yet the men were remarkably healthy; and among the causes of this health, Chisholm states that the necessary abstinence from strong liquors was one."

"In 1800 an English army, proceeding from India to Egypt to join Sir Ralph Abercromby, marched across the desert from Kossier, on the Red Sea, and descended the Nile for 400 miles. Sir James McGrigor says that the fatigue of this march has perhaps never been exceeded by any army, and goes on to remark: 'We receive still further confirmation of the very great influence which intemperance has as a cause of disease. We had demonstration how very little spirits are required in a hot climate to enable a soldier to bear fatigue, and how necessary a regular diet is. At Ghenné, and on the voyage down the Nile (on account of the difficulties of at first conveying it across the desert), the men had no spirits delivered out to them, and I am convinced that from this not only did they not suffer, but that it even contributed to the uncommon degree of health which they at this time enjoyed. From two boats the soldiers one day strayed into a village, where the Arabs gave them as much of the spirit which they distil from the juice of the date-tree as induced a kind of furious delirium. It was remarked that for three months after a considerable number of these men were in the hospitals.' "

The late Inspector-General Sir John Hall says :—
" My opinion is that neither spirit, wine, nor malt liquor
is necessary for health. The healthiest army I ever
served with had not a single drop of any of them ; and
although it was exposed to all the hardships of Kaffir
warfare at the Cape of Good Hope, in wet and inclement
weather, without tents or shelter of any kind, the sick
list seldom exceeded one per cent. ; and this continued
not only through the whole of the active operations in
the field during the campaign, but after the men were
collected in standing camps at its termination. And
this favourable state of things continued until the termination of the war. But immediately the men were
again quartered in towns and fixed posts, where they
had free access to spirits—an inferior species of brandy
sold there, technically called ' Cape Smoke '—numerous
complaints made their appearance among them."

The experience of lumbermen in the back-woods of
Canada has taught them the danger of indulgence in
alcohol when the cold is intense, and therefore during
the winter they are strict abstainers.

In advanced life, or in certain feeble conditions of
digestion, a moderate quantity of whiskey and water,
brandy and water, wine, or beer, may be useful and
advisable at meals ; but it should never be taken on an
empty stomach, nor early in the day. The greatest

quantity of absolute alcohol which an average man can take daily without injury to his health has been estimated at one ounce and a half. This is equivalent to about one wine-glass of rum, or to about one wine-glass and a half of brandy or whiskey, or to about four wine-glasses of sherry, port, Maderia, or Marsala, or to about one pint of Burgundy, claret, hock, or champagne, or to about two pints of beer.

The moral, social, and physical evils of intemperance are universally recognised. " Nor does anyone entertain a moment's doubt that the effect of intemperance in any alcoholic beverage is to cause premature old age, to produce or predispose to numerous diseases, and to lessen the chance of living very greatly." (Parkes.) The following figures, taken from Neison's vital statistics, may prove of interest.

In intemperate persons the mortality at twenty-one to thirty years of age is five times that of the temperate; from thirty to forty it is four times as great.

A temperate person's chance of living is	An intemperate person's chance of living is
At 20 = 44·2 years	At 20 = 15·6 years
,, 30 = 36·6 ,,	,, 30 = 13·8 ,,
,, 40 = 28·8 ,,	,, 40 = 11·6 ,,
,, 50 = 21·25 ,,	,, 50 = 10·8 ,,
,, 60 = 14·285,,	,, 60 = 8·9 ,,

Tobacco is a stimulant and restorative which, if used in moderation, soothes nervous irritability, allays hunger, and helps men to endure privations. Its effects are due to an active principle called *nicotine*, which is a powerful poison, and produces symptoms the opposite to those caused by *strychnine*, but equally fatal. When smoking is carried to excess, it produces tremors of the muscles, weakens the heart's action, and impairs the sight.

Moderation depends not only on the strength of the tobacco, but on the constitution of the smoker; and, as with everything else, one man may consume without injury what would be almost fatal to another. Smoking is a most pernicious habit in boys; it checks their physical as well as their mental development. No youth should touch tobacco before the age of twenty-three.

SECTION VII.

EXERCISE AND SLEEP.

In accordance with an admirable law which prevails in Nature, muscles increase (within certain bounds) in size, power, and fitness, in proportion to the amount of exertion which they are called upon to make. If the exertion be not carried to excess, all other parts of the body share in the beneficial effects; the lungs expand more fully, and the amount of air inspired and of carbonic acid expired is enormously increased; the heart acquires new vigour, sending the blood with greater force into all parts of the system; the digestive functions are carried on with increased activity, a higher degree of health ensues; and the intellect (if at the same time cultivated) becomes sound and active.

Whilst over-exertion should be carefully avoided, disuse of the voluntary muscles is followed by wasting and feebleness of the body generally. A judicious amount of exercise is therefore essential to a vigorous and healthy existence. The following valuable rules for the regulation of physical exercise are laid down by Dr. Cathcart :—

(1) It should be conducted in an abundance of fresh air, and in costumes allowing free play to the lungs, and of a material which will absorb the moisture, and which, therefore, should be afterwards changed—flannel.

(2) There should be a pleasant variety in the exercise, and an active mental stimulus, to give interest at the same time.

(3) The exercises should, as far as possible, involve all parts of the body, and both sides equally.

(4) When severe in character, the exercises should be begun gradually and pursued systematically, leaving off at first as soon as fatigue is felt ; and when any real delicacy exists, the exercise should be regulated under medical advice.

(5) For young people, the times of physical and mental work should alternate, and for the former the best part of the day should be selected.

(6) Active exertion should be neither immediately before nor immediately after a full meal.

History teaches us that gymnastics were practised by the ancient Greeks, not only with the view to military efficiency, but as the best means of obtaining a robust habit of body, and through it a vigorous intellect. In such estimation were they held for this purpose, that both Plato and Aristotle thought that no republic could be considered perfect in which gymnasia did not form part of the national institutions.

Nor did they estimate their value too highly, for it is now generally recognised that "the first requisite to success in life is to be a good animal, and to be a nation of good animals is the first condition of national prosperity." On the Continent, especially in Germany and Sweden, considerable attention is being paid to the best methods of promoting the physical development of the people.

Fortunately for England, sports and pastimes have always been a feature in the character of the nation, and this feature, judiciously trained and cultivated, is an important element of national greatness.

Field sports—hunting, shooting, fishing, etc.—not only supply the prime necessities of exercise and recreation, but tend to the formation of qualities which are in the highest degree useful in life—self-reliance, coolness, presence of mind, endurance, and fertility in resources.

Athletics may be regarded as including those manly games and pastimes which have been encouraged by all high-minded nations as calculated to develop and invigorate the bodily powers of their people.

Walking develops the muscles of the trunk and legs, increases the breathing power of the lungs, and improves the appetite and digestion. It is the most available means of obtaining healthy exercise, and is a useful adjunct to other forms of exercise, especially rowing.

Running, jumping, and throwing heavy weights are severe forms of exercise, and ought not to be undertaken without previous training and practice.

Cricket is the most popular of English games, and has come to be regarded as a pastime of national importance to the health and physique of the people. The activity, quickness of hand and eye, self-reliance, decision, and sound emulation which the game of cricket calls forth are productive of much good.

Rowing is a healthy and pleasant means of obtaining exercise. The muscles employed are chiefly those of shoulders, arms, and back, and to a less extent those of the lower limbs. It is largely indulged in by the students of Oxford and Cambridge, and has been found to be attended by the best results.

Swimming is one of the most invigorating forms of recreation ; it exercises almost all the muscles of the body, and cleanses the skin. It is the duty of every young person to learn to swim.

Polo, football, rackets, lawn-tennis, golf, and hockey are all admirable and popular games, and well adapted as a means of training body and mind for the battle of life.

Riding is a pleasant and exhilarating exercise,

suitable to all periods of life, from childhood to old age.   The beneficial effects of horse exercise on a "sluggish liver" has given rise to the saying that "the outside of a horse is the best thing for the inside of a man."

Although the above forms of exercise may be sufficient for those who can take advantage of them, yet there is a vast and increasing section of the community to whom sports and pastimes are almost unknown.   For this class, a course of training, such as men receive in the army, would be of inestimable value.

In addition to his military drills, &c., the recruit goes through a three months' course of gymnastic training, which often results in a pale and feeble youth being transformed into a robust and powerful man.   The good effects of gymnastics are well exemplified in the case of twelve non-commissioned officers who were trained as gymnastic instructors for the army by Mr. McLaren, of the Oxford Gymnasium.   The men ranged from 19 to 29 years of age, and in height from 5 feet 5 in. to 6 feet. In Mr. McLaren's own words :—" The muscular additions to the arms and shoulders and the expansion of the chest were so great as to have absolutely a ludicrous and embarrassing result, for before the fourth month several of the men could not get into their uniform jackets and tunics without assistance, and when they got them on, they could not get them to meet by a hand's breadth. In a month more they could not get into them at all, and new clothing had to be procured, pending the arrival of which the men had to go to and from the gymnasium in their great-coats. One of these men had gained five inches in actual girth of chest." Mr. McLaren goes on to say:—"There was the change in bodily activity, dexterity, presence of mind, and endurance of fatigue: a change a hundred-fold more impressive than anything the tape measure or the weighing-machine can ever reveal."

It is difficult to determine the actual amount of exercise which a healthy adult should take; but the following facts are sufficiently established for practical purposes. A moderate day's work is generally taken at 300 foot tons, a hard day's work at 450, and a very hard day's work at 600. A certain time must be allowed for this work, as velocity increases its exhausting effects; or, in other words, "It is the pace that kills." Fifty foot tons an hour is considered a fair amount, and this rate is equal to a walk of three miles on a level road.

Professor Haughton has calculated that walking on a level surface is equivalent to raising 1-20th part of the weight of the body through the distance walked. "Using this formula," says Professor Parkes, "and assuming a man to weigh 150 lbs. with his clothes, we get the following table :—

Kind of Exercise.									Work done in Tons lifted one foot.
Walking 1 mile	.	.	.	.	.	.	.		17·67
,, 2 ,,	.	.	.	.	.	.	.		35·34
,, 10 ,,	.	.	.	.	.	.	.		176·7
,, 20 ,,	.	.	.	.	.	.	.		353·4
,, 1 ,, and carrying 60 lbs.			.	.	.				24·75
,, 2 ,, ,, ,,			.	.	.	.			49·5
,, 10 ,, ,, ,,			.	.	.	.			247·5
,, 20 ,, ,, ,,			.	.	.	.			495

"Looking at all these results," he continues, "and considering that the most healthy life is that of a man engaged in manual labour in the free air, and that the daily work will probably average from 250 to 350 tons lifted 1 foot, we can perhaps say, as an approximation, that every healthy man ought, if possible, to take a daily amount of exercise in some way which shall not be less than 150 tons lifted 1 foot. This amount is equivalent to a walk of about nine miles; but then, as there is much exertion taken in ordinary business of life, this amount may be in many cases reduced."

Man is said to be a low-pressure engine, working all his organs considerably under their full power. In the case of exercise, the amount required for the purposes of health is far short of that which can be accomplished by men in good training and condition.

The following instances of long marches during war may be interesting, as well as instructive :—

"The 43rd, 52nd, and 95th Regiments of Foot, forming the Light Division under Crawfurd, made a forced march in July, 1809, in Spain, in order to reinforce Sir Arthur Wellesley at the battle of Talavera. About fifty weakly men were left behind, and the brigade then marched sixty-two miles in twenty-six hours, carrying arms, ammunition, and pack—in all, a weight between 50 lbs. and 60 lbs. There were only seventeen stragglers.

"One of these regiments—the 52nd—made in India, in 1857, a march nearly as extraordinary. In the height of the mutiny, intelligence reached them of the locality of the rebels from Sealkote. The 52nd and some artillery started at night on the 10th of July, 1857, from Umritzur, and reached Goodasepore, forty-two miles off, in twenty hours, some part of the march being in the sun. On the following morning they marched ten miles, and engaged the mutineers. They were for the first time clad in the comfortable grey or dust-coloured native Kharki cloth.

"A company of a regiment of Chasseurs of Mac-Mahon's army, after being on grand guard, without shelter or fire, during the rainy nights of the 5th-6th August, 1870, started at three in the morning to re-join its regiment in retreat on Neiderbronn, after the battle of Weissenburg. It arrived at this village at 3.30 in the afternoon, and started again for Phalsbourg at 6 o'clock. The road was across the hills and along forest tracks, which were very difficult for troops. It arrived at Phals-bourg at 8.30 o'clock in the evening of the next day. The men had, therefore, marched part of the night of the 5th-6th August, the day of the 6th, the night of the 6th-7th, and the day of the 7th till 8.30 p.m. The halts were eight minutes every hour from 3.30 to 6, one hour in the night of the 6th-7th, and 2½ hours on the 7th. Altogether, including the halts, the march lasted 41½ hours, and the men must have been actually on their feet about thirty hours, in addition to the guard duty on the night before the march.

"An officer of a Saxon Fusilier Regiment gave the following statement of a forced march in one of the actions at Metz in 1870. The regiment was alarmed at midnight, and marched at 1 a.m., and continued marching, with halts, until 7 p.m.; they bivouacked for the night, marched at 7 the next morning, came into action at 1.30, and in the evening found themselves 15 kilomètres beyond the field of battle. The total dis-tance was 53½ miles in forty-two hours, with probably 15 hours' halt.

"Roth mentions that the 18th Division of the Saxon

army in the various manœuvres about Orleans marched, on the 16th and 17th of December, 1870, 54 English miles.

"Von der Tann's Bavarian army, in retreat on Orleans, marched 42 miles in twenty-six hours.

"After Sedan, the Prussian and Saxon troops pushed on to Paris by forced marches, and accomplished, on an average, 35 kilomètres, or 21⅔ miles, daily, and they marched on some days 42 to 45 kilomètres (26 to 28 miles). They started at five or six, and were on their ground from four to eight o'clock, the average pace being 5 kilomètres (3·1 miles) per hour.

"In the Indian Mutiny several regiments marched 30 miles a day for several days."

It should be observed that the larger the body of men, the slower the march. A single regiment can do 20 miles in eight hours, but a large army will take twelve or fourteen, including halts. (Parkes.)

SLEEP.

Sleep is that period of repose, or rest, which is requisite for the renewal of the muscular and nervous energy which active exertion tends to exhaust. Different individuals and ages require different amounts of sleep. The popular idea that a child sleeps half its time, an adult one-third, whilst an old person may do little

except eat and sleep, is near the truth.   Seven or eight
hours is usually ample for healthy adults, with nine
hours on Sundays.   Some men can do with much less:
for instance, Sir George Elliot, who commanded at the
great siege of Gibraltar, never slept more than four hours
in the twenty-four during the siege, which lasted nearly
four years.

SECTION VIII.

CLOTHING.

THE chief object of clothing is to protect the body against hurtful variations of cold and heat, with as little restraint upon the movements of the limbs and the action of the internal organs as possible.

For protection against cold, wool is much superior, weight for weight, to either cotton or linen. Its capacity for absorbing moisture renders it most suitable for under-clothing, especially after exertion, when it prevents too rapid cooling of the body. Merino, which is a mixture with twenty to fifty per cent. of wool, is light and porous, and well adapted for under-clothing in hot climates. It is less liable than flannel to deteriorate—shrink and become hard—by frequent washing.*

For protection against cold winds and rain, leather and indiarubber fabrics, according to Dr. Parkes, take the first rank, wool the second, and cotton and linen

---

* In washing woollen articles, they should never be *rubbed* or *wrung*. They should be placed in a hot solution of soap, moved about, and then plunged into cold water. When the soap is got rid of, they should be hung up to dry without wringing. (Parkes.)

F

the last. Waterproof clothing is, however, unsuited for constant wear, as it retains and condenses the perspiration.

As a protection against excessive solar heat, the texture of clothes has little influence; this depends chiefly, if not entirely, on colour. White has the greatest protecting power; then grey, yellow, pink, red, blue, black. For hot climates, therefore, white or grey clothing should be chosen.

As regards the garments themselves. "Everything," says Dr. Parkes, "should be as simple and effective as possible; utility, comfort, durability, and facility of repair are the principles which should regulate all else."

The popular advice to "keep the feet warm and the head cool" is a sound maxim, and should be carefully carried out. The head-dress should be light, well ventilated, and impervious to rain; it should fit easily, and not press on the head. A heavy head-dress is apt to produce a sense of oppression, and to diminish the supply of blood going to the scalp. The actual weight of certain head-dresses may be interesting.

The tall black hat weighs 7 ozs., the Infantry helmet 14½ ozs., the Hussar busby 29¾ ozs., the Lancer cap 34½ ozs., the bearskin 37 ozs., the helmet of the heavy Dragoons 39 ozs., and the helmet of the Cavalry of the Guard 55 ozs.

The boots should be of such a size and shape as to allow of the free expansion of the foot during the act of walking; the inner line of the boot should be straight, so as not to push the great toe outwards. The soles should be flexible and impervious to wet; the heels low and broad, for the purpose of giving firm support to the weight of the body. A perfectly rigid sole prevents the foot from exerting its natural spring and action, and tends to cause wasting of the muscles of the leg. * Boots or shoes that are made too narrow at the toes are liable to produce corns, bunions, and in-growing toe-nails. Professor Koch, in a lecture delivered at Berlin in 1888, stated that at the beginning of the last war, 30,000 men were made useless for service owing to unsuitable foot-gear.

* A pair of light shoes might, with advantage, be substituted for the extra pair of ankle boots which the soldier carries in his pack. (R. C. E.).

SECTION IX.

CLIMATE.

By climate is understood the combined effect of heat, moisture, atmosphere, wind, soil, and electrical conditions in their relation to animal and vegetable life.

The human body seems to have a marvellous power of adapting itself to varying climatic conditions; and it may be accepted as a general principle that, so long as reasonable care is observed, a healthy man can live and flourish on almost any part of the earth's surface.

Much of the sickness that was formerly attributed to climate is known now to be really due to local insanitary conditions.

"Take away these sanitary defects," says Dr. Parkes, "and avoid malarious soils, or drain them, and let the mode of living be a proper one, and the European soldier does not die faster in the tropics than at home."

The soil or site on which a dwelling is built has considerable influence on the health of the inhabitants. Dry and permeable soils, such as gravel, sand, and chalk, or those which have such a slope as to allow of natural drainage, are healthy; on the other hand, flat, moist, and alluvial soils are unhealthy. Soils containing much organic matter are to be avoided, such as those made in towns from rubbish of all sorts, as well as marshy districts.

The air in soils is almost always impure, hence the necessity for covering the site on which a dwelling is to be placed with a layer of concrete or other impermeable material, so as to prevent the *ground-air* from rising within the house.

At varying depths below the surface there exists a subterranean sheet of water, known as *ground* or *sub-soil water*, which is in constant movement, in most cases flowing towards the nearest water-courses or the sea. Much importance is attached to it; and Professor Von Pettenkofer lays down that a permanently high ground water—that is, within five feet of the surface—is bad, while a permanently low ground water—that is, more than fifteen feet from the surface—is good.

Vegetation, as a rule, has a beneficial influence on soils. In cold climates, trees shelter from the cold winds, but they obstruct the passage of the sun's rays to the soil, thus rendering it liable to be cold and damp.

In hot climates, trees shade the ground and make it cooler, whilst the evaporation from the leaves lowers the temperature of the air and tends to dry the soil. It has been found that the evaporation from an oak-tree during the summer was 8⅓ times the rain-fall; and observations in Algeria have shown that the blue gum-tree absorbs and evaporates 11 times the rain-fall. Herbage is always healthy; in the tropics it shades the ground from the direct rays of the sun, and tends to cool and equalise the temperature.

In dense forests there is generally an accumulation of decaying vegetable matter, which, under the influence of heat, moisture, and stagnant air, is productive of malarial fevers.

Brushwood is objectionable in the neighbourhood of dwellings, and should be removed.

In selecting a site for habitations, a dry, porous soil should be chosen: in an elevated position, if available, and on a gentle slope favourable to free drainage. Hollows or enclosed valleys should be avoided, as well as positions in close proximity to the foot of hills.

Dr. Parkes gives the following five conditions as requisite to ensure healthy habitations:—

(1) A site dry, and not malarious, and an aspect which gives light and cheerfulness.

(2) A system of ventilation which carries off all respiratory impurities.

(3) A system of immediate and perfect sewage

removal, which shall render it impossible that the air shall be contaminated from excreta.

(4) A pure supply and proper removal of water; by means of which perfect cleanliness of all parts of the house can be ensured.

(5) A condition of house construction which shall ensure perfect dryness of the foundation, walls, and roof.

SECTION X.

PREVENTION OF DISEASE.

THE best means of preventing disease is to be found in a careful and loyal obedience to established sanitary principles, as laid down with reference to cleanliness, pure air, pure water, proper food and drink, good drainage, and unpolluted soils. Such precautions are preventive of malarial fevers, cholera, enteric fever, yellow fever, typhus, dysentery, diphtheria, erysipelas, lung diseases, &c.

Small-pox is guarded against by vaccination and re-vaccination. The primary operation should be performed within four or six weeks after birth, and repeated after the fourteenth year. The evidence as to the efficacy of vaccination is very conclusive. " In the Franco-German war, which took place in the great epidemic years 1870-72, small-pox was introduced into the French army by the Breton recruits, and carried off 23,000 men ; while the Germans, who followed on their track, and had, moreover, charge of most of their sick, but who, if not vaccinated in childhood, were so on enlistment, lost only 226." Dr. Collie, in " Quain's Dictionary of Medicine," says :—" It may be stated generally that the unvaccinated will die at the rate of 50 per cent., the badly vaccinated at the rate of 26 per cent., and the well vaccinated at the rate of about 2·3 per cent."

In the case of scarlet fever and measles, a good sanitary condition lessens their severity, and isolation arrests their spread.

During the Middle Ages frightful epidemics of plague, sweating sickness, and other diseases, visited this country at frequent intervals, and caused immense mortality. It has been stated that in 1348 half the population of England perished of plague alone. The epidemic swept over the whole of Europe, killing about twenty-six millions of people, " and the ravages were fiercest in the greater towns, where filth and undrained streets afforded a constant haunt for leprosy and fever."

In London, from 1660 to 1670—a period in which the plague was prevalent—the death rate was 80 per 1,000. But when the worst plague-spots—the small, overcrowded, and filthy houses in the metropolis—were destroyed by the Great Fire, the disease became less severe. This led to increased attention being paid to the demands of sanitary science, and since then the death rate of London has gradually diminished. At the beginning of the nineteenth century it had fallen to 29 per 1,000; in 1840-49 it was 25·3 ; in 1870-78 it was 23 ; and at the present time it is under 20. This

remarkable decrease in the mortality is, undoubtedly, due
to the enormous sanitary improvements which have been
carried out in the city during the present century.

"Whoever," says Dr. Parkes, "considers carefully the
record of the mediæval epidemics, and seeks to interpret
them by our present knowledge of the causes of disease,
will surely become convinced that one great reason why
those epidemics were so frequent and so fatal was the
compression of the population in faulty habitations. Ill-
contrived and closely-packed houses, with narrow streets,
often made winding for the purposes of defence ; a very
poor supply of water, and therefore a universal uncleanli-
ness ; a want of all appliances for the removal of excreta ;
a population of rude, careless, and gross habits, living
often on innutritious food, and frequently exposed to
famine from their imperfect system of tillage—such
were the conditions which almost throughout the whole
of Europe enabled diseases to attain a range and to
display a virulence of which we have now scarcely a con-
ception. The more these matters are examined, the
more shall we be convinced that we must look, not to
grand cosmical conditions ; not to earthquakes, comets,
or mysterious waves of an unseen and poisonous air ;
not to recondite epidemic constitutions, but to simple,
familiar, and household conditions, to explain the spread
and fatality of the mediæval plagues."

In former campaigns it was reckoned that for one man who was killed in battle six died from diseases, such as typhus fever, cholera, dysentery, &c. During the first winter, 1854-55, in the Crimea, the average strength was 31,333, and the losses from disease 10,285 ; in the second winter, 1855-56, the average strength was 50,166, and the losses from disease only 551. This wonderful change in the rate of mortality was due to the labours of the Army Sanitary Commission, which was sent out to the Crimea in the spring of 1855. The beneficial results achieved by this Commission, as well as the practical lessons in sanitary science taught by Crimean experience, are well described in the " History of the United States Sanitary Commission," from which the following brief extracts are taken :—

"At that time the experience of the Crimean War was fresh in the memory of all. That experience was a complete chapter by itself on Sanitary Science. It taught the great truth that the ' cause of humanity was identified with the strength of armies.' We were left in no vague conjecture as to the causes which produced the fearful mortality among the allied troops before Sebastopol—a mortality which, as has been truly said, has never been equalled since the hosts of Sennacherib fell in a single night. Public opinion in England, indignant and horror-stricken at this frightful result, long

before the war closed, called loudly for investigation and
remedy.   The result has been a contribution of inestimable value to our knowledge of everything which
concerns the vital questions of the health, comfort, and
efficiency of armies.

   " The experience of the Crimean War taught those
who consulted it the nature of the terrible dangers
which encompass all armies outside of the battle-field,
the possibility of mitigating them, and the sanitary
measures which, in strict accordance with the general
laws of health, should be adopted to provide for the
safety of an army.

   " The importance, therefore, of rousing public opinion
to the absolute necessity of forcing upon the Government the adoption of precautionary measures to ensure
the lives and safety of our troops in camps, in barracks,
and in hospitals, was the practical lesson which was
taught by the Crimean experience of those who had
studied it, with a view to rendering it applicable to
our needs.

   " The powers conferred on the British Sanitary
Commission were wholly unexampled in the history
of the administrative system of Great Britain.   The
results of its labours have been, on the whole, perhaps
the grandest contribution ever made by Science to the
practical art of preserving health among men required

to live together in large masses. Its existence was due, as we have said, to the horror which was inspired by the accounts of the perishing army before Sebastopol, and to the widespread conviction that this result was attributable to causes which might be removed by wise sanitary measures. Three gentlemen, each distinguished for his practical acquaintance with the laws of Hygiene and the principles of Sanitary Science—Dr. Sutherland, Dr. Hector Gavin, and Mr. Rawlinson *—were appointed in February, 1855, by the Minister of War, Lord Panmure, commissioners to proceed at once to the Crimea (subsequently, on the death of Dr. Gavin, Dr. Milroy was appointed), and there, on the spot, to reform the abuses to which the evil was due."

Again, Dr. J. N. Radcliffe, in " The Hygiene of the Turkish Army," writes :—" The cleanliness of a camp is a subject of peculiar importance, and the methods of attaining cleanliness merit more attention than they have yet received on the part of military officers.

" Cleanliness, so far as the neat aspect of a camp is concerned, is highly gratifying to the eye ; but this may be, and indeed often is, attained, and yet some of the worst sources of atmospheric pollution, from a misapprehension of their effects, are allowed to remain.

" The continued inhalation of an atmosphere tainted

* Now Sir Robert Rawlinson, C.B.

by decomposing organic matter, such as is usually rife in a camp, is one of the most powerful predisposing causes of those terrible epidemics which ravage armies. It insidiously deteriorates the health, and lays the foundation necessary for the development of fever, cholera, and other cognate diseases; and inasmuch as it is less palpable in its effects than bad diet, excessive fatigue, intemperance, and other potent predisposing causes of disease, which are apt to affect an army in the field; and as it is more generally—nay, is invariably—present in a greater or less degree, it requires more constant and watchful attention. Remove the predisposing causes of an epidemic disease, and the exciting cause becomes, as a rule, inoperative; diminish the former in degree, and the latter will be proportionately diminished in effect. For many years the experience of civil life has shown that the emanations from decomposing substances act most powerfully in predisposing the system to the development of fever, dysentery, diarrhœa, and cholera. The experience of the allied armies during the war in the Crimea has shown that in the camp the effluvia from putrescent matters were equally powerful agents in the development of diseases among the soldiers, and that the diseases thus developed were similar in character to those witnessed under the same circumstances in civil life.

" To diminish the sources of atmospheric vitiation in a camp, it is requisite that proper receptacles should be provided for all ejected matters whatsoever; that it should be imperative upon the soldier to use these receptacles; that measures should be had recourse to for the destruction of such rejected matters as cannot be readily and deeply buried; that a systematic watchfulness should be observed on the part of the officers; and that special regulations should be adopted for the guidance of the men. Nothing can be done effectually without a properly organised scheme of action, equally affecting the superior and inferior grades of officers and the men. The sanitary state of a camp is a matter of too great importance to admit of the measures necessary to secure the conditions most favourable to the preservation of health being left to the option of one man or another.

" Not unfrequently the site of an encampment was insufficiently prepared, the drainage in particular being defective; and when the soil happened to be naturally moist, the air within the tents was rendered damp, and this condition operated as a powerful localising cause of zymotic disease."*

Vast improvements have been made in army sanitation since the Crimean War; and the errors and

* " The Hygiene of Armies in the Field," by Sir Robert Rawlinson, C.B.

mal-arrangements of former times are now corrected—
or, at least, the means of correcting them are known.

It remains for the soldier to realise how much he
has within his own power, as regards his well-being and
physical happiness.

Professor Huxley says :—" Knowledge of Nature is a
guide to practical conduct. Anyone who tries to live
upon the face of this earth without attention to the laws
of Nature will live there for but a very short time, most
of which will be passed in exceeding discomfort; a
peculiarity of natural laws, as distinguished from those
of human enactment, being that they take effect without summons or prosecutions."

An effort has been made in the preceding pages to
inculcate a knowledge of the laws of life and health,
whereby men may be enabled to live in comfort, and to
maintain their bodies in a condition not only free from
disease, but full of energy, strength, and endurance ; and
from these results they may learn to look upon sanitary
regulations not "as mere commands based on no particular grounds," but as rules founded on the noblest of
all sciences—the Science of Health.

Printed by Cassell & Company, Limited, La Belle Sauvage, London, E.C.

Printed in the United States
By Bookmasters